ABC OF AIDS

Fourth edition

ABC OF AIDS

Fourth edition

edited by

MICHAEL W ADLER MD FRCP

Professor of Genitourinary Medicine, University College and Middlesex School of Medicine

with contributions by

C A AITKEN, PETER BEVERLEY, R P BRETTLE, KEVIN M DE COCK, LESLEY FRENCH, ROB GEORGE, DI GIBB, JONATHAN GRIMSHAW, CAROLINE GUINNESS, MICHAEL HARRISON, M HELBERT, D J JEFFRIES, ANNE JOHNSON, IAN MCGOWAN, DAVID MILLER, ROB MILLER, ADRIAN MINDEL, P P MORTIMER, PAUL ROGERS, MARGARET SPITTLE, NINA SWIRE, MELINDA TENANT-FLOWERS, GARETH TUDOR-WILLIAMS, IAN V D WELLER, IAN WILLIAMS

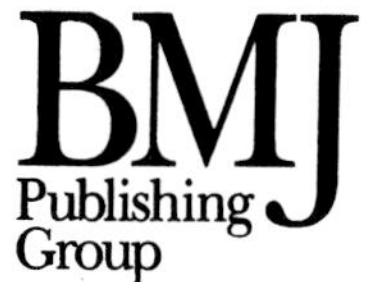

First edition 1987
Second impression 1987
Third impression 1988
Fourth impression 1988
Fifth impression 1990
Second edition 1991
Third edition 1993
Fourth edition 1997

British Library Cataloguing in Publication Data

ISBN 0-7279-1137-6

Typeset by Apek Typesetters Ltd., Nailsea, Bristol
Printed and bound by Craft Print, Singapore

Contents

INTRODUCTION

By September 1996 there were 13 400 patients with AIDS in the UK and 28 000 screened and infected with HIV. Many of those with the virus are well, asymptomatic, and even unaware that they are infected, but others, although they have not yet developed AIDS, have physical, psychological, social and occupational problems and require as much care as those with AIDS. We therefore need to be concerned not with "a few cases" but with a large number of people infected with the virus, who will be making demands on every part of the health and social services. New infections will occur, and the public health education campaign will need to continue. None of us should feel that the problem of HIV infection and AIDS is unimportant and that it will go away because of the campaign and the possible magic bullet of a cure or vaccine.

We can all hope for these things but it would be a mistake to be lulled into a state of inertia and complacency. All of us will be concerned with AIDS for the rest of our professional lives. This book, originally written as weekly articles for the *BMJ*, attempts to give those doctors and other health care workers, who currently have had little experience of AIDS and HIV, some idea of the clinical, psychological, social, and health education problems that they will become increasingly concerned with.

Patients with HIV and AIDS remain well for long periods. The median incubation period from infection to AIDS is estimated to be eight to nine years and may be longer, and once diagnosed patients can live for several years. Once a patient develops AIDS an acute illness will demand admission to hospital. Once these illnesses start to occur the patient usually recovers but at each supervening illness becomes a little weaker. Currently we believe that up to 80% of people infected with HIV will develop AIDS, but this proportion has changed since the early days and may continue to change. The range of infection with HIV is wide: totally well asymptomatic individuals who make limited demands on services; those with chronic infection, shown by chronic skin and other infections; and those with full blown AIDS, who make heavier demands.

Patients with HIV infection and AIDS spend most of their time out of hospital in the community. Admission is required only when an acute clinical illness supervenes. General practitioners and domiciliary and social services do not always feel skilled and knowledgeable enough to look after them. With the increase in the number of cases, the community services will have to be able and willing to cope. Again, I hope that this book will help to make people feel more skilled and comfortable about caring for patients with HIV and AIDS.

A variety of approaches can be adopted for looking after patients with varying degrees of HIV infection and AIDS. Providing such care is a challenge for all of us. I have no doubt that we will respond to that challenge and will be able to look back and know that we tried and showed the same commitment and dedication to this problem as to all others that we face each day. None of us should adopt a rigid and uncaring stance towards patients with HIV infection and AIDS; that might mean we look back at our professional lives with a feeling of shame rather than one of endeavour and, I hope, achievement.

This is the fourth edition of the *ABC of AIDS*; each chapter has been updated or rewritten and new chapters on Palliative care and pain control, and Having AIDS added.

Michael W Adler

1 DEVELOPMENT OF THE EPIDEMIC

Michael W Adler

History of the epidemic

1981 Cases of *Pneumocystis carinii* pneumonia and Kaposi's sarcoma in the United States

1983 Discovery of the virus. First cases of AIDS in the United Kingdom

1984 Development of antibody test

AIDS-defining conditions without laboratory evidence of HIV

- Diseases diagnosed definitively
  - Candidiasis: oesophagus, trachea, bronchi or lungs
  - Cryptococcosis: extrapulmonary
  - Cryptosporidiosis with diarrhoea persisting >1 month
  - Cytomegalovirus disease other than in liver, spleen, nodes
  - Herpes simplex virus (HSV) infection
    - mucocutaneous ulceration lasting >1 month
    - pulmonary, oesophageal involvement
  - Kaposi's sarcoma in patient <60 years of age
  - Primary cerebral lymphoma in patient <60 years of age
  - Lymphoid interstitial pneumonia in child <13 years of age
  - *Mycobacterium avium*: disseminated
  - *Mycobacterium kansasii*: disseminated
  - *Pneumocystis carinii* pneumonia
  - Progressive multifocal leukoencephalopathy
  - Cerebral toxoplasmosis

The first recognised cases of the acquired immune deficiency syndrome (AIDS) occurred in the summer of 1981 in America. Reports began to appear of *Pneumocystis carinii* pneumonia and Kaposi's sarcoma in young men, who it was subsequently realised were both homosexual and immunocompromised. Even though the condition became known early on as AIDS, its cause and modes of transmission were not immediately obvious. The virus now known to cause AIDS in a proportion of those infected was discovered in 1983 and given various names. The internationally accepted term is now the human immunodeficiency virus (HIV). Subsequently a new variant has been isolated in patients with West African connections—HIV-2.

The definition of AIDS has changed over the years as a result of an increasing appreciation of the wide spectrum of clinical manifestations of infection with HIV. Currently, AIDS is defined as an illness characterised by one or more indicator diseases. In the absence of another cause of immune deficiency and without laboratory evidence of HIV infection (if the patient has not been tested or the results are inconclusive), certain diseases when definitively diagnosed are indicative of AIDS. Also, regardless of the presence of other causes of immune deficiency, if there is laboratory evidence of HIV infection, other indicator diseases that require a definitive, or in some cases only a presumptive, diagnosis also constitute a diagnosis of AIDS.

In 1993 the Centers for Disease Control (CDC) in the United States of America (USA) extended the definition of AIDS to include all persons who are severely immunosuppressed (a CD4 count $<200 \times 10^6$/l) irrespective of the presence or absence of an indicator disease. For surveillance purposes this definition has not been accepted within the UK and Europe. In these countries AIDS continues to be a clinical diagnosis defined by one or more of the indicator diseases mentioned. The World Health Organisation (WHO) also uses this clinically based definition for surveillance within developed countries. WHO, however, has developed an alternative case definition for use in sub-Saharan Africa (see chapter 10). This is based on clinical signs and does not require laboratory confirmation of infection. Subsequently this definition has been modified to include a positive test for HIV antibody.

AIDS-defining conditions with laboratory evidence of HIV

- Diseases diagnosed definitively
  - Recurrent/multiple bacterial infections in child <13 years of age
  - Coccidiomycosis-disseminated
  - HIV encephalopathy
  - Histoplasmosis-disseminated
  - Isosporiasis with diarrhoea persisting >1 month
  - Kaposi's sarcoma at any age
  - Primary cerebral lymphoma at any age
  - Non-Hodgkin's lymphoma: diffuse, undifferentiated B cell type, or unknown phenotype
  - Any disseminated mycobacterial disease other than *M. tuberculosis*
  - Mycobacterial tuberculosis at any site
  - Salmonella septicaemia: recurrent
  - HIV wasting syndrome
  - Recurrent pneumonia within 1 year
  - Invasive cervical cancer
- Diseases diagnosed presumptively
  - Candidiasis: oesophagus
  - Cytomegalovirus retinitis with visual loss
  - Kaposi's sarcoma
  - Mycobacterial disease (acid-fast bacilli; species not identified by culture): disseminated
  - *Pneumocystis carinii* pneumonia
  - Cerebral toxoplasmosis

CDC Definition of AIDS

Effective 1 January 1993:
All those with confirmed HIV infection with CD4 T lymphocyte count $<0{\cdot}2\times10^6$/l
± indicator disease

These case definitions are complex and any clinician who is unfamiliar with diagnosing AIDS should study the documents describing them in detail.

Transmission of the virus

Transmission of the Virus

- Sexual intercourse
  - anal and vaginal
- Contaminated needles
  - intravenous drug users
  - needlestick injuries
  - injections
- Mother → child
  - *in utero*
  - at birth
  - breast milk
- Organ/tissue donation
  - semen
  - kidneys
  - skin, bone marrow, corneas, heart valves, tendons etc.

HIV has been isolated from semen, cervical secretions, lymphocytes, cell-free plasma, cerebrospinal fluid, tears, saliva, urine, and breast milk. This does not mean, however, that these fluids all transmit infection since the concentration of virus in them varies considerably. Particularly infectious are semen, blood, and possibly cervical secretions. The commonest mode of transmission of the virus throughout the world is by sexual intercourse. Whether this is anal or vaginal is unimportant. Other methods of transmission are through the receipt of infected blood or blood products, donated organs, and semen. Transmission also occurs through the sharing or reuse of contaminated needles by injecting drug users or for therapeutic procedures, and from mother to child. Transmission from mother to child occurs *in utero* and also possibly at birth. Finally, the virus is transmitted through breast milk.

HIV Transmission: Global Summary

Type of exposure	Percentage of global total
Blood transfusion	3–5
Perinatal	5–10
Sexual intercourse	70–80
(vaginal)	(60–70)
(anal)	(5–10)
Injecting drug use (sharing needles, etc.)	5–10
Health care (needlestick injury, etc.)	<0·01

There is no well documented evidence that the virus is spread by saliva. It is not spread by casual or social contact. Health care workers can, however, be infected through needlestick injuries, and skin and mucosal exposure to infected blood or body fluids. Prospective studies in health care workers suffering percutaneous exposure to a known HIV seropositive patient indicate a transmission rate of 0·32%. As of December 1995 there have been 79 reported cases of documented seroconversion after occupational exposure in such workers.

The precautions and risks for such groups are covered in detail in chapter 15. Finally, there is no evidence that the virus is spread by mosquitoes, lice, bed bugs, in swimming pools, or by sharing cups, eating and cooking utensils, toilets, and air space with an infected individual. Hence, HIV infection and AIDS are not contagious.

Growth and size of the epidemic

Even though North America and Europe experienced the first impact of the epidemic, infections with HIV are now seen throughout the world, and the focus of the epidemic is in developing/resource-poor countries.

Cumulative AIDS cases reported to the World Health Organisation, June 1996

The Americas	690 042
Europe	167 578
Africa	499 037
Oceania	7 285
Asia	29 707
Total	1 393 649

Worldwide

By June 1996, 1 393 649 cumulative cases of AIDS had been reported in children and adults throughout the world. This is thought to be a considerable underestimate, particularly from continents such as Africa, and WHO estimate that the real total is 7·7 million cases. WHO have also estimated a cumulative total of 27·9 million HIV infections since the start of the epidemic (25·5 in adults and 2·4 in children), and that this will rise to 30–40 million infections by the year 2000.

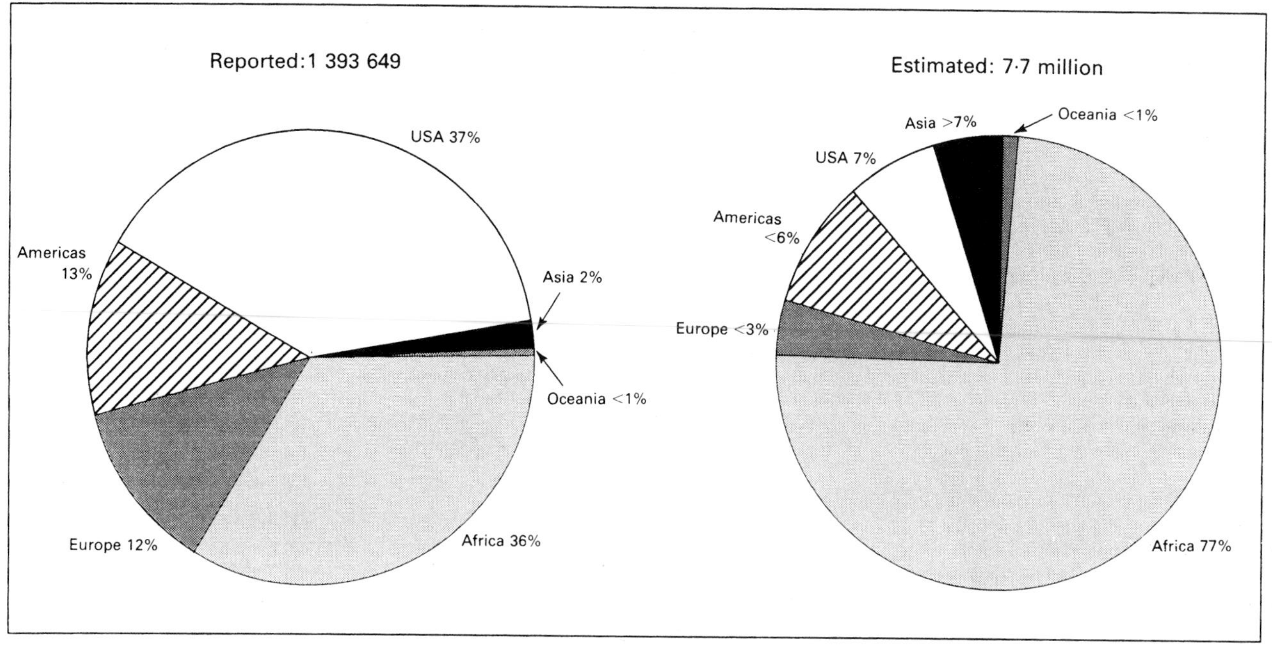

Total cumulative number of AIDS cases in adults and children from late 1970s/early 1980s until mid 1996.

Epidemiological characteristics of AIDS: sub-Saharan Africa compared to United Kingdom and United States

Characteristic	Sub-Saharan Africa	UK/USA
Homosexuality	Little or none	50–75% of all cases
Intravenous drug user	Little or none	6–25% of all cases
Heterosexual transmission	Very common	Less common
Male to female	1:1	1:7–10
Other concurrent STDs	Frequently documented	Documented less often

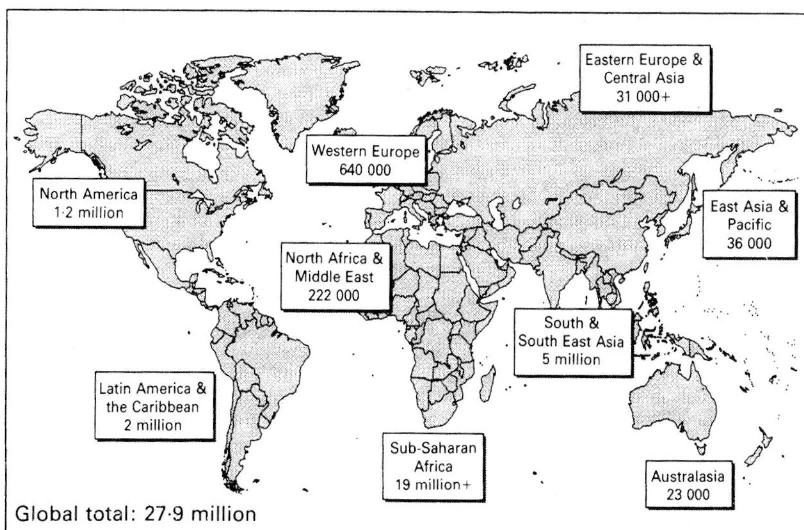

Estimated distribution of total HIV infections from late 1970s/early 1980s until mid-1996.

Currently, 80% of all infections occur in developing countries and continents, the major brunt of the epidemic being seen in sub-Saharan Africa and south-east Asia. One in fifty adults is infected in Thailand, one in forty in sub-Saharan Africa, and in some African countries, this figure runs as high as one in three adults. It is now recognised that cases of AIDS were first seen in Central Africa in the 1970s even though at that time it was not recognised as such. Current surveys from some African countries show that the prevalence of infection is high amongst certain groups—50–90% of prostitutes, 30% of those attending departments for sexually transmitted diseases and antenatal clinics.

In the developing world, HIV is spread mainly by heterosexual intercourse and the male to female ratio of infection is virtually 1:1. Studies of heterosexual transmission have shown different rates of transmission, with the female partners of men with HIV and AIDS showing the highest rates of approximately 25%. Transmission from infected women to their male partners is lower at about 10%.

The demographic, economic, and social impact of AIDS is far reaching with considerable effects on individuals, families, and countries. At a family level, WHO estimates up to 15 million uninfected children in Africa will have lost their mothers to AIDS by the end of the century. Traditional family structures and extended families are breaking down under the strain of HIV. Population growth and death rates will be increasingly affected. There is a marked reduction in life expectancy due to AIDS in most developing countries. Young highly productive adults die at the peak of their output, which has a considerable impact on a country's economy.

AIDS—Adult patient groups in USA and UK, June 1996

	USA		UK	
Patient groups	No	%	No	%
Men who have sex with men	274 192	51	9 344	73
Intravenous drug user	137 753	25	782	6
Men who have sex with men and I.V. drug user	35 218	7	—	—
Haemophilia	4 280	1	584	5
Received blood	7 684	1	126	1
Heterosexual contact	44 980	8	1 812	14
Other/undetermined	36 699	7	132	1
Total	540 806	100	12 780	100

United States, United Kingdom and Europe

By June 1996, 540 806 adult cases had been reported in the USA. AIDS is now the major cause of premature death in young men. Also, by the end of 1996 there was an additional 7 296 paediatric cases (<13 years old). Most (90%) of the cases in children occur because a parent suffered from HIV or belonged to a group at increased risk of HIV; 5% occurred through blood transfusion; 3% in children with haemophilia. Information on risk factors for the remaining 2% of parents of these children is not complete.

Adult cases in Europe totalled 168 163 by June 1996, and those in the UK 12 780. There are five times more people infected with HIV at any one time than have AIDS. The rate for AIDS cases varies throughout Europe, with particularly high rates in Italy, Spain, France, and Switzerland, where the commonest mode of infection is through intravenous drug use and the sharing of needles and equipment.

HIV-1 infections and AIDS cases: UK to end 1996
Sex between men and women

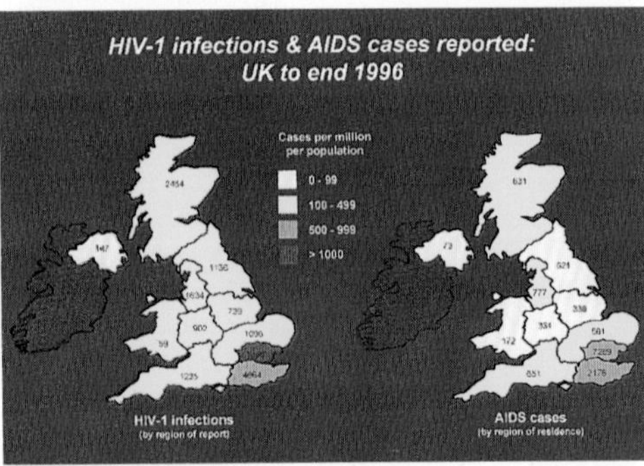

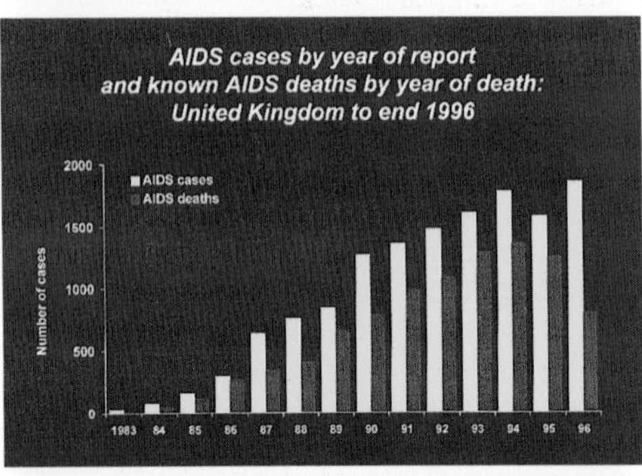

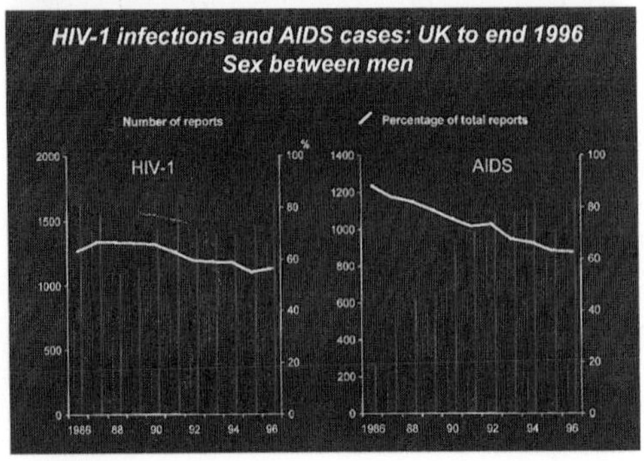

In North America and the UK the first wave of the epidemic occurred in homosexual men. In the UK, proportionally more homosexual men have been notified than in America: 73% of cases compared with 51% respectively. Even though infections amongst men who have sex with men still arise, an increasing proportion of new infections in the USA is occurring amongst intravenous drug users sharing needles and equipment. There is also an increase amongst heterosexuals in both the USA and the UK. Currently in the USA, 14% of cases of AIDS have occurred amongst women, and although the commonest risk factor amongst such women is injecting drug use (46%), the next most common mode of transmission is heterosexual contact (38%).

The nature of the epidemic within the UK is changing with more heterosexual transmission. In the UK 10% of adult cases of AIDS have occurred in women, two thirds of which have resulted from heterosexual intercourse. Up to 1985, 2% of all HIV infections had resulted from sexual intercourse between men and women; by mid 1996 this had risen to 30%. Recent results from anonymous seroprevalence studies among pregnant women in inner London show levels of infection as high as 0·5% in some districts, and for men and women attending clinics for sexually transmitted diseases in the capital, levels of 1·5% and 0·6% respectively have been shown. Infections amongst drug users and gay men have slowed down, but still occur. Of particular concern is the level of new infections among young gay men in London, which is still high.

Relation between the virus and the disease

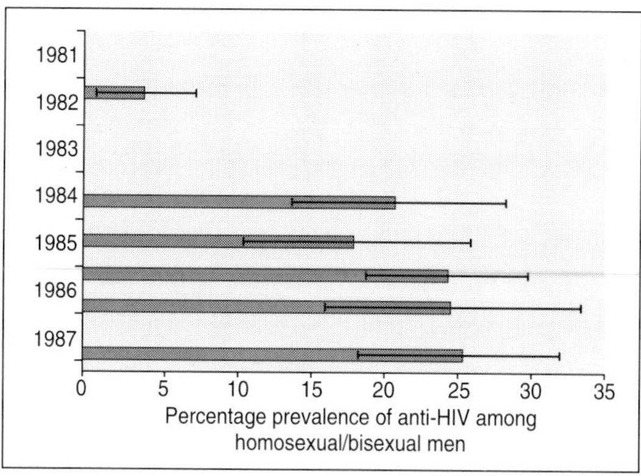

Prevalence of anti-HIV in men attending the Middlesex Hospital, London, during 1981–87. (Bars are 95% confidence limits.)

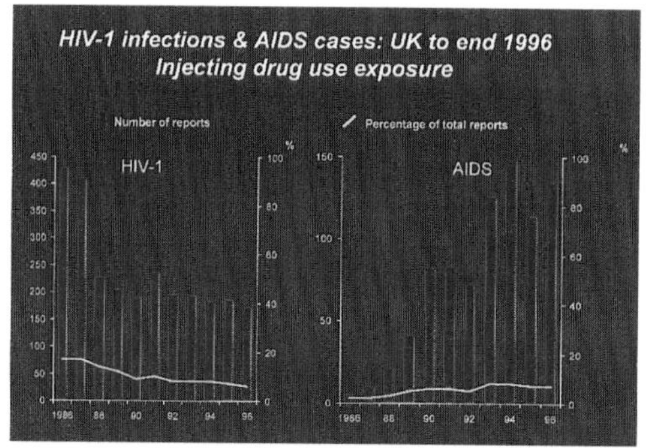

The advent of an effective antibody test in 1984 has allowed for a clearer understanding of the changing prevalence and natural history of HIV infection. For example, tests on stored samples of serum collected for other reasons from a cohort of homosexual men in San Francisco give an indication of how the epidemic evolved. In 1978, 4% were anti-HIV positive; by 1980 the proportion had increased sixfold, to 24%. In British provincial centres and especially London the rate of seropositivity has increased in a similar fashion. These surveys show that the proportion of individuals infected needs to be high before cases of AIDS start to become apparent. It also underlines the importance of health education campaigns early in the epidemic, when the seroprevalence of HIV is low. Once cases of AIDS start to appear the epidemic drives itself and a much greater effort is required in terms of control and medical care.

The rate of infection has also increased in other groups. In Southern Italy the prevalence of HIV antibody among intravenous drug users increased from below 1% in 1980 to 76% in 1985. Similar large increases among drug users have been seen in European countries such as Switzerland, Spain, and Italy.

Within countries one finds considerable variation in seroprevalence levels for HIV. Over 70% of cases of AIDS and HIV infection within the UK occur and are seen in the Thames regions (London and the surrounding area). Among different groups one also finds geographical differences. For example, the rates among drug users is higher in Edinburgh than London, and for gay men higher in London than anywhere else in the UK. This is also found in the developing world; for example, in Tanzania and Uganda, the urban level of HIV infection in men and women can be five times higher than rural rates.

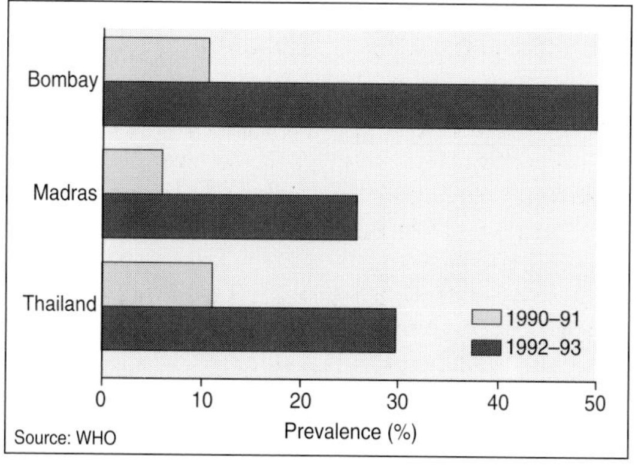

HIV prevalence in female prostitutes, Asia 1990–93.

In the developing world, the same rapid increase in HIV prevalences is seen as in developed countries. Thus, marked increases over short periods of time have been seen among prostitutes in India and Thailand, and in drug users in south/south-east Asia.

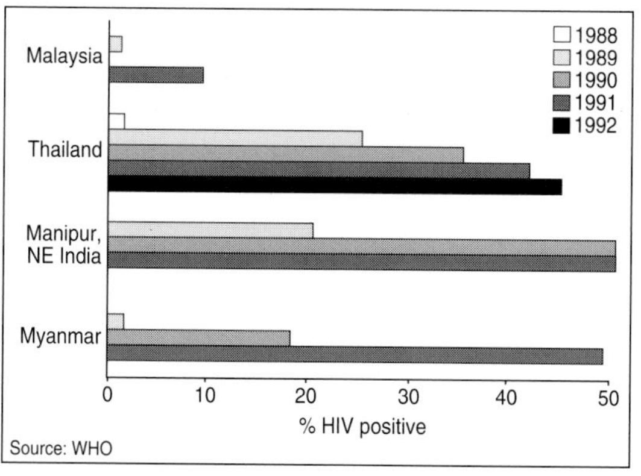

HIV prevalence in injecting drug users in south/south-east Asia 1988–92.

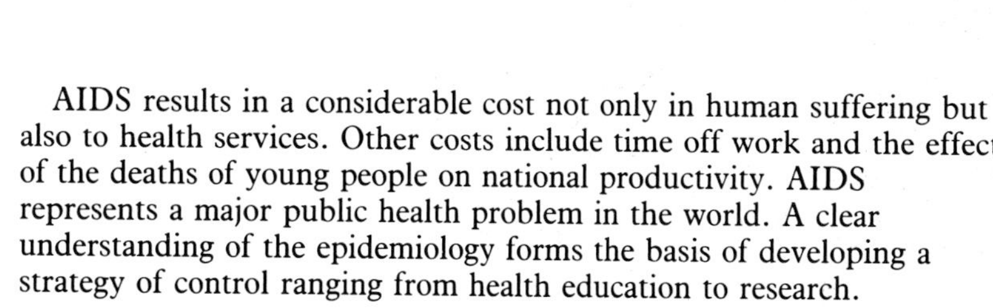

AIDS results in a considerable cost not only in human suffering but also to health services. Other costs include time off work and the effect of the deaths of young people on national productivity. AIDS represents a major public health problem in the world. A clear understanding of the epidemiology forms the basis of developing a strategy of control ranging from health education to research.

2 THE VIRUS AND THE TESTS

P P Mortimer

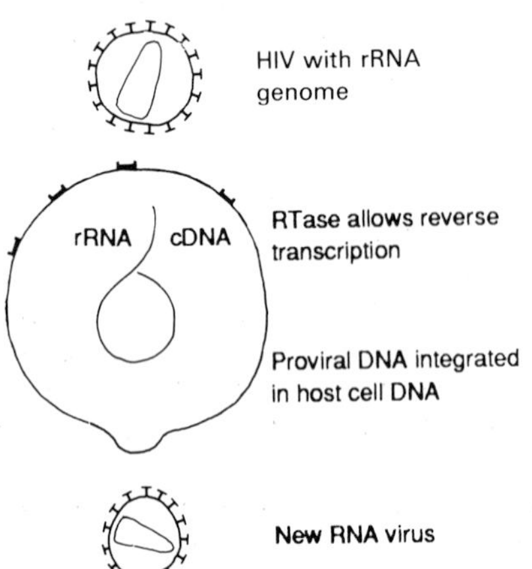

Although it is clear that HIV is the underlying cause of AIDS and AIDS-related disease, its origin remains obscure. There is a firm serological evidence of infection on the east and west coasts of the USA from the mid-1970s, and HIV infection in central Africa may have antedated infection in North America, but there is as yet no proof. It is possible that phylogenic analysis of HIV subtypes, including observations of the rate at which mutations arise in subtypes, will soon throw more light on the emergence of HIV-1. In the case of HIV-2, the similarity to the simian virus SIV may point to an animal origin, as may also be the case for HIV-1. Like some other RNA viruses, HIV is very labile, and consequent shifts in host range and virulence would explain how a new pathogenic retrovirus could arise in man. Alternatively, HIV may have existed as a latent, mainly vertically transmitted infection in a sequestered human population for very many years and its virulence may have recently been amplified as a result of travel, population dislocation, and promiscuous sexual contact, with rapid passage of the virus.

Retroviruses are so named because their genomes encode an unusual enzyme, reverse transcriptase, which allows DNA to be transcribed from RNA. Thus HIV can make copies of its own genome, as DNA, in host cells such as the human CD4 "helper" lymphocyte. The viral DNA becomes integrated in the lymphocyte genome, and this is the basis for chronic HIV infection. This integration of the HIV genome into host cells is likely to be a formidable obstacle to the development of any antiviral agent that would not just suppress but also eradicate the infection. The inherent variability of the HIV genome and the failure of the human host to produce neutralising antibodies to the virus, as well as technical difficulties and concerns about safety, continue to frustrate attempts to make an effective vaccine.

A particular concern is that a vaccine developed in North America or Europe against the locally prevalent HIV-1 subtype will be ineffective in those parts of the world where other subtypes predominate. It must be conceded that the mass of data that has accumulated about the lineage of HIV in the last decade has seemed only to show how hard it is to explain the origin of HIV and how difficult it may be to eradicate it now that it is established in most continents. In 1996, WHO estimates suggest that there were nearly 27·9 million cumulative cases of HIV worldwide since the start of the epidemic.

HIV and related viruses

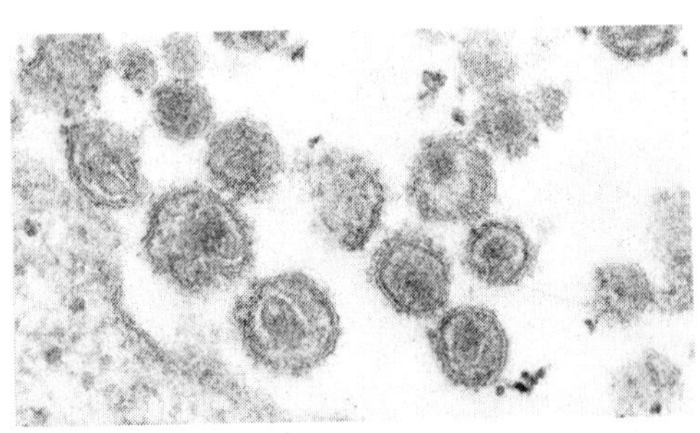

HIV particles, many showing typical lentivirus morphology (× 100 000).

HIV was discovered by Barré-Sinoussi, Montagnier, and colleagues at the Institut Pasteur, Paris, in 1983 and given the name lymphadenopathy associated virus (LAV). In 1984 Popovic, Gallo, and coworkers described the development of cell lines permanently and productively infected with the virus and, in line with two previously described retroviruses, HTLV-I and HTLV-II, they designated the virus HTLV-III, LAV, HTLV-III. Other viruses since isolated from patients with AIDS and AIDS-related disease in America, Europe, and Central Africa are all the same virus, and this is the virus now referred to as HIV-1. At least six subtypes of HIV-1, alphabetically designated, have now been described.

Around 1985 another retrovirus, different from HIV-1, was recognised in patients with West African connections. This virus, referred to by the Paris investigators as LAV-2 and more recently as HIV-2, is also associated with human AIDS and AIDS-related disease, though it is more closely related to a simian retrovirus, SIV, carried by healthy African green monkeys, than it is to HIV-1. SIV causes an AIDS-like disease in captive rhesus monkeys. Though potentially important worldwide, HIV-2 infections are uncommon outside West Africa.

Nomenclature of human retroviruses

(a) Two lentiviruses causing AIDS, HIV-1 (previously LAV, HTLV-III) with six major subtypes A–F, and outliers, HIV-10 and HIV-2

(b) Two oncoviruses causing lymphoma and leukaemia
HTLV-I
HTLV-II

Transmission of HIV infection

HIV-1 and HIV-2, the major and minor human AIDS viruses, are transmitted in ways that are typical for all retroviruses—"vertically", that is from mother to infant, and "horizontally" through sexual intercourse and through infected blood. At certain times carriers of HIV probably excrete much more virus than others. These periods can be recognised by measuring the p24 antigen in blood or quantifying viral DNA or RNA (see below). Transmission also depends on other factors, such as trauma, secondary infection, the efficiency of epithelial barriers, the presence or absence of cells with receptors for HIV, and perhaps the immune competence of the exposed person. All infections with HIV seem to become chronic and some have been shown to be continuously productive of virus. The ultimate risk of spread to those repeatedly exposed is therefore high.

Transmission factors

- Phase of infection
- Virus titre
- Trauma
- Secondary infection
- Epithelial damage
- Intensity of exposure

The stage of infection is an important determinant of infectivity. In most virus infections the highest titres of virus are reached early in infection, before antibody is produced. For HIV this phase is difficult to study because symptoms are mild or non-existent and the anti-HIV response undetectable; nevertheless, it is a time when an individual is very likely to infect contacts. There is also evidence that when, much later, AIDS supervenes the individual again becomes highly infectious. In the long interval between there may be periods when, except through massive exposures—for example, blood donation—infected individuals are virtually non-infectious. In the absence of reliable quantifiable markers of infectivity, however, all seropositive individuals must be seen as potentially infectious, and effective but humane ways found to protect their contacts in cases where risk arises. This has led to the promulgation of the concept of "safe sex" which should inform sexual contact between all individuals regardless of whether they are known to be infected with HIV.

Tests for anti-HIV-1 and -2

Anti-HIV

- Appears 3 weeks to 3 months after exposure
- Has weak neutralising capacity

Three ways of detecting anti-HIV

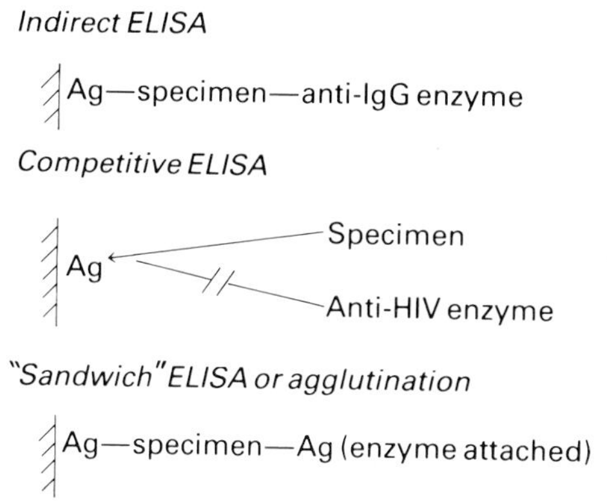

Indirect ELISA

Ag—specimen—anti-IgG enzyme

Competitive ELISA

Ag ← Specimen
Ag ← // — Anti-HIV enzyme

"Sandwich" ELISA or agglutination

Ag—specimen—Ag (enzyme attached)

Anti-HIV tests have transformed our understanding of the epidemiology of AIDS in the years since they were introduced in 1984, and are still the bedrock of diagnosis and much preventive and epidemiological research. Anti-HIV appears three weeks to three months after exposure to HIV and thereafter is invariably detectable in spite of any detrimental effect the virus may have on lymphocyte function and antibody production. It has been suggested that a long interval may sometimes occur between exposure to infection and the antibody response, but this seems to be very unusual indeed, and there is no evidence of infectivity during that time. Though neutralising antibodies to HIV are measurable, their titres are low and their effect weak. They do not obviously limit the progress of infection and disease. Inability to mount a neutralising response to HIV antigens is the most likely reason why conventional approaches to preparing a vaccine will fail.

At first HIV was prepared from cell lines in large amounts for diagnostic purposes, then purified, and used as an antigen in serological tests. However, similar antigens can now be made by DNA cloning and expression or by synthesis of viral polypeptides. Several types of anti-HIV test exist, and three that are available commercially are illustrated. Most tests use an enzyme conjugate and give a colour signal due to the

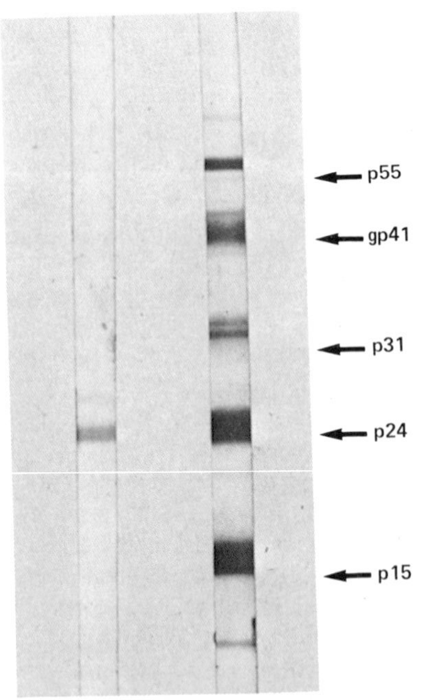

The left strip, a Western blot result from a serum specimen collected soon after HIV infection, shows antibody to p24 without other bands being clearly visible. The right strip, a result on a serum sample collected from the same patient 3 months later, shows antibody to many viral proteins, including p15, p24, p31, gp41, and p55.

reaction between an enzyme specifically bound to antigens on a polystyrene surface, membrane or inert particles and a substrate; other tests depend on the binding of a fluorescein or chemiluminescent conjugate, or the visible agglutination of HIV-coated gelatin or latex particles.

Since anti-HIV tests became commercially available in 1985 they have been widely used in diagnostic and transfusion laboratories in the developed world. The accuracy—both sensitivity and specificity—of the antibody assays is continually being improved, and the occurrence of false positive and false negative results is probably less and less frequent. The proportion of true to false positive results depends on the population studied, but even in low risk groups such as blood donors it is now very high in well conducted laboratories. Human errors cause most false results. The key to avoiding these mistakes is continuous review with repeat testing where necessary. Ideally, all positive reactions should both be confirmed by additional assays and succeeded by tests on a follow up specimen (see below). The use of several screening tests in parallel on proven positive specimens also acts as a check on false negativity in screening assays (which it is otherwise difficult to guard against).

Modern screening kits detect antibody to both HIV-1 and HIV-2. Anti-HIV-2 is mostly encountered in West Africans and Europeans who have lived in west Africa. It has also been reported on the Indian subcontinent, but is very rare in the Americas. In the United Kingdom blood donations and clinical specimens are now routinely tested for both HIV-1 and HIV-2 infection.

In addition to methods for detecting "whole" anti-HIV, the more discriminating tests recognise components of the antibody response. The serological response to individual HIV proteins can be studied by Western blot and the immunoglobulin class response in blood and other fluids can also be investigated. The IgM response slightly precedes the IgG response early in infection. The IgA response is a feature of infection in infancy.

Simple tests, confirmatory tests, follow-up tests

Simpler anti-HIV screening tests have been developed for large scale testing in unfavourable laboratory conditions and when results are needed urgently—for instance, before transplantation procedures. Saliva and urine can conveniently be used as specimens to investigate for anti-HIV when venepuncture is difficult. Simple and rapid tests and non-invasive tests are attractive options and will allow developments such as home testing, but few are as accurate as the conventional assays on serum, and checks such as follow-up confirmatory tests are essential before a positive diagnosis is made by these means.

In many countries, including the United Kingdom, procedures have been introduced to secure accurate testing. The most important is that when there is a positive anti-HIV finding the test is repeated and the implicated specimen is tested by other, methodologically independent, anti-HIV assays. Another specimen should then be sought. Although this may lead to some delay in confirming positive findings, anti-HIV results are as a consequence much more precise. The greatest remaining anxieties are that a few infected individuals may either not have anti-HIV when tested or have it in such low concentrations that even sensitive assays fail to detect it; or that there has been technical or clerical error. Follow up at an interval of one to four weeks is often a valuable diagnostic expedient, as well as greatly diminishing the chances of either false negative or false positive anti-HIV results. The most important element in the successful laboratory diagnosis of HIV infection is indeed access to follow-up specimens. When newly infected individuals are followed up, the titre and range of HIV antibodies usually increases and those who have been infected for several months or more almost invariably have strong anti-HIV reactions. Persistently weak anti-HIV reactions are usually non-specific. Sometimes PCR (see below) will resolve a difficult-to-confirm reactive specimen. Correct follow-up procedures also guard against specimen misidentification and transcription errors.

Tests for the virus: antigen, viral DNA and RNA

Viral antigens are detectable in serum, in particular the HIV core antigen p24. This is detectable only for so long as it is in excess of antibody to p24, typically at the outset of infection. Tests for this HIV antigen are commercially available, and they assist in the diagnosis of early infection and the recognition of infection in infants. In more advanced infection the presence of HIV antigen and of other non-specific markers of increased viral replication implies immune deterioration and may be an indication for antiviral treatment. In practice, tests for HIV antigen have proved of limited value due to a lack of sensitivity although this may be enhanced by acid or alkali dissociation of immune complexes in the specimen before it is assayed for p24.

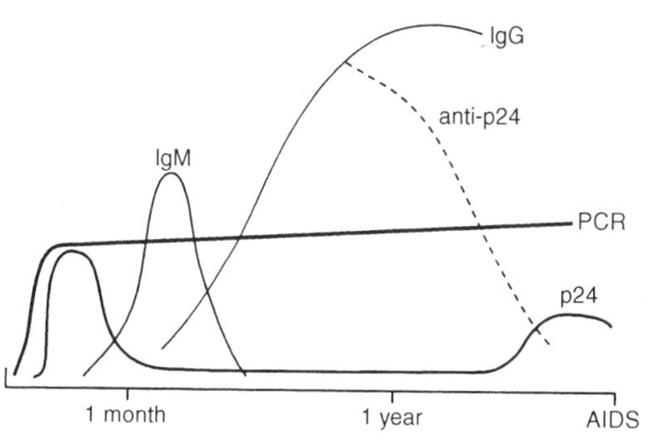

Viraemia, recognised by isolation of HIV from plasma, is demonstrable even in the presence of high titres of anti-p24 and antibodies to other HIV proteins. However, virus isolation is time consuming and essentially a research tool.

HIV can also be recognised in specimens as genome sequences. Only rare lymphocytes carry HIV genome, but the polymerase chain reaction can be used greatly to amplify chosen HIV genome sequences in clinical specimens containing only small numbers of infected lymphocytes. To a large extent viral culture has been superseded by this PCR amplification of HIV DNA extracted from mononuclear cells in the circulation, and by reverse transcription and amplification of HIV RNA also present in blood. Though these procedures are less accurate than anti-HIV assays and more expensive, they are useful in diagnosis in infancy when the anti-HIV detected may be of maternal origin. They also provide rapid access to the HIV genome and therefore characterisation of an HIV isolate to strain level. Also within reach is (semi)quantification of viraemia which is likely to become an important determinant of treatment, especially as the choice of antiviral combinations widens. Targets for genome amplification include the genes coding the main envelope and core proteins. On the basis, particularly, of analysis of sequences of amplified sections of the envelope gene, HIV-1 has been subtyped—HIV subtypes A to F. In some cases the sequences found in the envelope and core genes are not concordant as, for example, strains of subtype B, suggesting that recombination may occur in HIV as it does, for instance, in influenza A virus. Sequencing of PCR "amplicons" is also the basis for analysis of HIV transmissions in special settings, for example, health care.

Testing of patients and blood donors

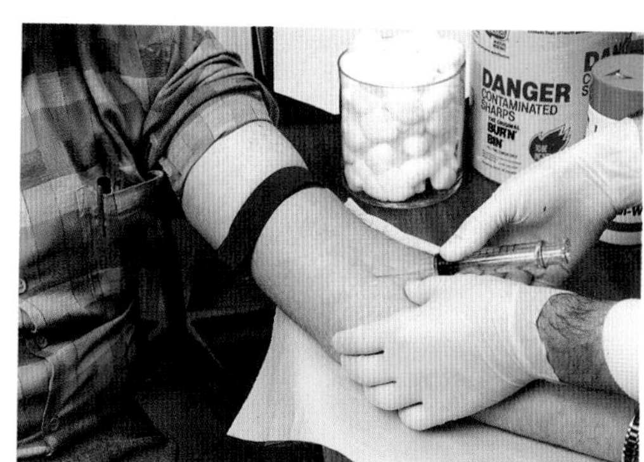

Tests for anti-HIV-1 and -2, HIV-1 antigen and HIV-1 genome are now widely available in the United Kingdom. Anti-HIV tests are done almost daily in most public health laboratories and are also in daily use in transfusion centres. The facilities in transfusion centres emphatically do not exist to provide testing for those at risk however. Indeed, the main means by which the blood supply is protected from contamination with HIV is through those individuals at increased risk of HIV infection refraining from giving blood (see Chapter 16).

Those who want to be tested for anti-HIV should instead consult their general practitioner or attend a sexually transmitted diseases (genitourinary medicine) clinic, where the advisability of HIV testing will be discussed. If a decision to test is made the necessary investigations are readily and freely available. In some localities "open access" facilities are being piloted to encourage responsible self-referral for counselling and testing. Other innovations, such as home testing on the patient's own initiative, are being considered in the USA and might be imported into the UK.

Kits with which people can test themselves are now technically feasible. It is important to be aware of the psychological impact of test findings on those who are being tested. While the emergence of effective drug treatment for HIV carriers is making widespread testing for anti-HIV a more attractive proposition there should be an element of medical supervision and it is debatable whether the telephone help lines that are proposed in support of home testing can provide this.

Important precautions

Taking and transporting specimen

Careful venepuncture (clotted blood)

Dispose of syringe and needle safely

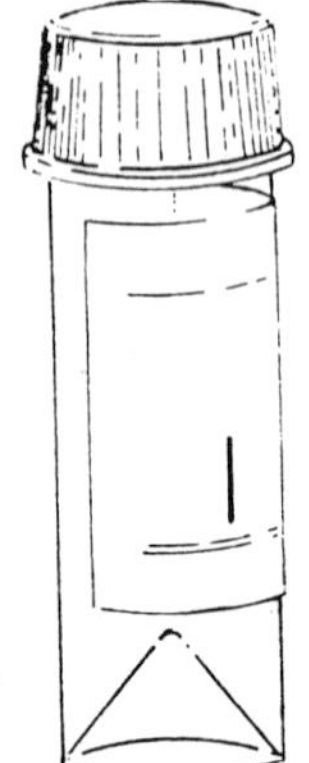

Place blood in a leakproof container that has a screw cap with rubber liner
Tighten firmly

Label specimen with patient's number and date of collection

Seal specimen in polythene bag, preferably using heat sealer, with request form attached outside

Send container to laboratory by secure route

Share information only with named staff in confidence

The need to discuss investigations for HIV infection with patients beforehand and to interpret the results to them afterwards is discussed elsewhere in this book. When named patients are tested for anti-HIV in a health care setting, permission to collect a sample should always have been sought by the doctor and expressed by the patient. An exception to this is when serum residues, irreversibly anonymised, are tested for anti-HIV as part of an epidemiological study. These studies have become the basis of the epidemic projections needed for prediction of the trends and for resource management. Clotted blood for testing should be obtained by careful venepuncture without spillage or risk of an inoculation accident. The needle and syringe should be disposed of safely and the blood placed in a leakproof container, properly identified, and sent by a secure route to the laboratory. PCR testing requires a fresh EDTA specimen.

The patient's identity and the suspected diagnosis should not be exposed to public gaze, so numbers or codes rather than names may have to be used, even though the risk of misidentification is increased. Patient information should be shared over the telephone only between individuals who know each other, and written reports should be sent to named members of staff in confidence, and under confidential cover. All positive results should be checked again on a freshly drawn specimen. The consequences of breaches of these procedures may be very serious for patients as well as damaging to the reputation and medicolegal position of doctors. Because of the implications of positive laboratory findings for the health of the patient, his or her family and contacts, and for the patient's social and professional life, a high level of competence and sensitivity is to be expected from all who are concerned in instigating investigations for HIV infection.

Laboratory tests for HIV have increased understanding of AIDS and greatly facilitated diagnosis, management, treatment, and control measures. However, to derive most benefit from them and do least harm they must be used wisely, with proper regard to all the possible consequences for those who are being tested. Any changes to what are now well established procedures must be carefully considered, piloted, evaluated for cost-effectiveness, and, if introduced, periodically audited to ensure that they are yielding the benefits promised.

The Western blot illustration was provided by J P Clewley and the electron micrography by J E Richmond.
The data on AIDS/HIV in the UK on pages 4 and 5 are reproduced with permission of CDSC.

3 IMMUNOLOGY OF AIDS

Peter Beverley, Matthew Helbert

Immunopathology

Many of the clinical features of HIV infection can be ascribed to the profound immune deficit which develops in infected individuals. HIV is immunosuppressive because it infects cells of the immune system and ultimately destroys them. An understanding of this process is helpful in interpreting tests used in monitoring the disease and may explain the failure of immunotherapy and the difficulties in developing vaccines for HIV.

The main target of the virus is a subset of thymus-derived (T) lymphocytes carrying the surface molecule CD4, which has been shown to bind the envelope glycoprotein of HIV (gp120). The destruction of CD4 lymphocytes accounts at least in part for the immunosuppressive effect of the virus.

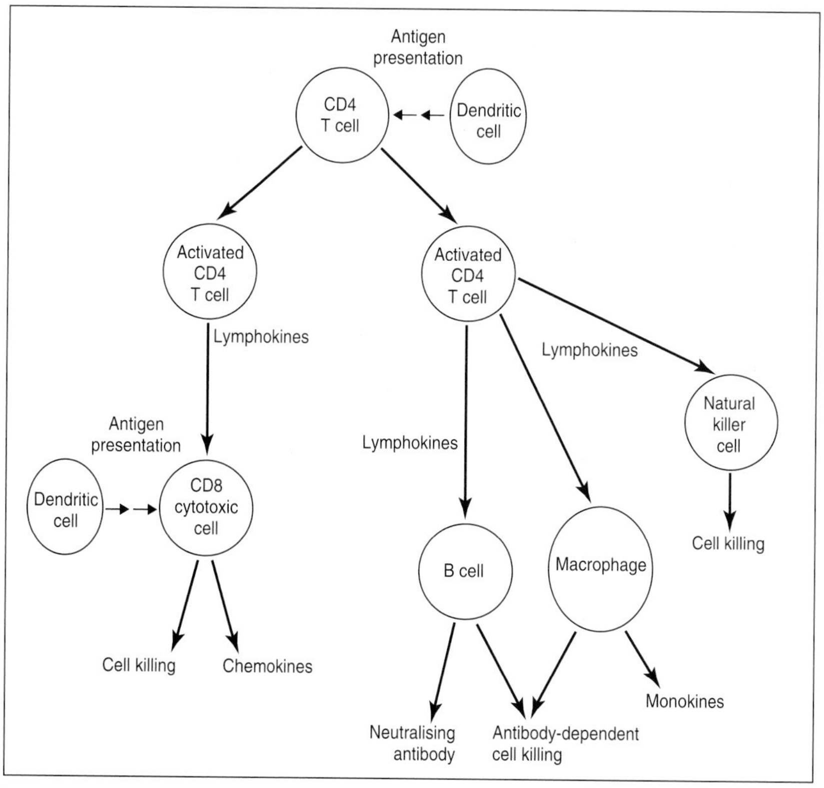

Induction of an immune response.

CD4 lymphocytes (T helper cells) have been termed "the leader of the immunological orchestra" because of their central role in the immune response. When these cells are stimulated by contact with an antigen they respond by cell division and the production of lymphokines, such as interferons, interleukins, tumour necrosis factor, and the chemoattractant chemokines. Lymphokines act as local hormones controlling the growth, maturation, and behaviour of other lymphocytes, particularly the cytotoxic/suppressor (CD8) T cells and antibody-producing B lymphocytes. Lymphokines also affect the maturation and function of monocytes and tissue macrophages.

In the early stages after HIV infection antibody responses are not impaired; indeed, development of antibodies to the virus envelope and core proteins is the principal evidence for HIV infection and persists until death. In adults, massive activation of B lymphocytes is manifested by a rise in serum immunoglobulin concentration, perhaps due to direct activation of B cells by HIV. This polyclonal activation explains why a variety of false positive serological tests are seen in HIV infection. In young children, the reverse pattern may be seen, with extremely low levels of immunoglobulin sometimes requiring intravenous replacement therapy.

It has now been recognised that CD4 is also present on a large proportion of monocytes and macrophages, Langerhans' cells of the skin, and dendritic cells of blood and lymph nodes. These cells are important antigen-presenting cells for initiating immune responses of lymphocytes. Not only do they act as a reservoir for the virus but their antigen-presenting function is impaired, with secondary effects on lymphocytes. Monocytes are the precursors to some glial cells, and abnormal lymphokine production after HIV infection may have harmful effects on neural tissue and result in HIV encephalopathy.

Within days or weeks after infection there may be a transient fall in CD4 lymphocyte numbers and a more sustained rise in the number of CD8 cytotoxic/suppressor cells. Among the CD8 cells, expanded

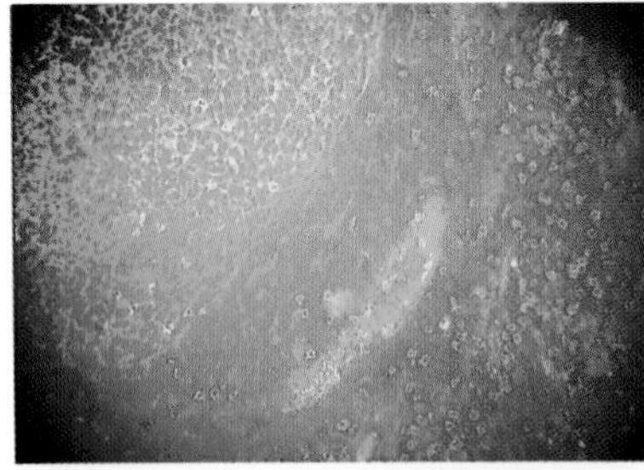

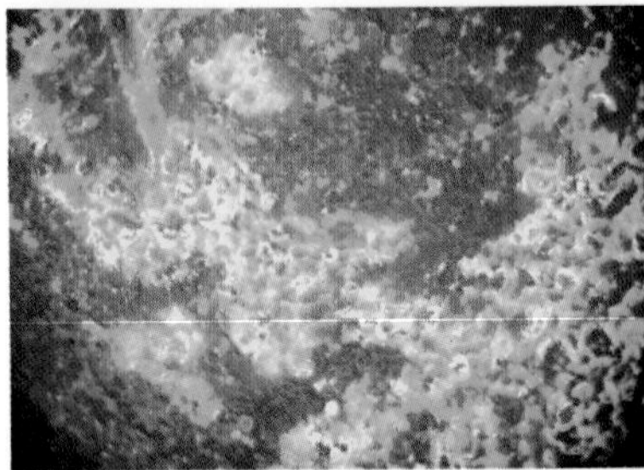

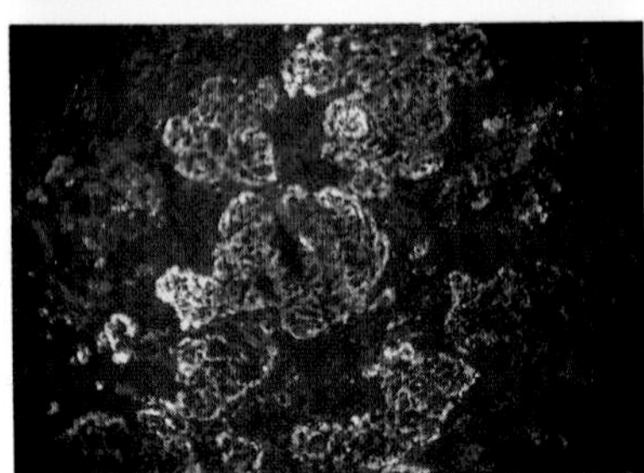

oligoclonal populations are frequently seen, but it is not yet clear whether these represent a specific response to HIV. Following this acute reaction, healthy seropositive individuals may have normal numbers of lymphocytes, although the numbers of CD8 cells frequently remain high. Even at this stage, however, *in vitro* testing may show a lowered response to previously encountered (recall) antigens (tetanus toxoid or purified protein derivative, for example). This seems to be due to poor production of the lymphokine interleukin 2. Individuals may remain healthy for long periods, but a hallmark of disease progression, often prior to the development of new clinical symptoms, is a fall in the number of CD4 lymphocytes. In AIDS the number of CD8 lymphocytes also falls.

Biopsy of the lymph nodes in patients with persistant generalised lymphadenopathy shows many enlarged follicles, often infiltrated by CD8 lymphocytes, with depletion of CD4 cells. Even in clinically silent HIV infection, lymph nodes are the site of remarkably active HIV replication. Uninfected cells may also die by apoptosis, initiated by unexplained mechanisms. In the later stages lymph nodes return to normal size and follicles become "burnt out", with loss of normal architecture and progressive cellular depletion.

Top: Normal lymph node in which B lymphocytes and follicular dendritic cells (green) form a regular network and suppressor/cytotoxic CD8 T cells (red) populate the paracortical areas. *Middle*: Node from HIV-positive patient with persistent generalised lymphadenopathy which has been infiltrated by many CD8 cells and in which the regular structure has been destroyed. *Bottom*: Same section as middle picture showing complexes of HIV core antigen (orange) and immunoglobulin (red) deposited in germinal centre.

Specific immune responses to HIV

In spite of the fact that HIV-infected individuals show the gross abnormalities of immune function described above, they are able to mount a specific immune response to HIV itself. Although serum reactivity to all the viral proteins is detectable, virus-neutralising titres are generally low and directed against the immunising virus strain (type-specific immunity). Passive transfer of antibody from asymptomatic to symptomatic patients is claimed to be beneficial but this requires confirmation. Antibodies to HIV may even facilitate infection of cells bearing immunoglobulin (Fc) receptors, such as monocytes. In AIDS a fall in the titre of antibodies to core protein (p24) is often associated with disease progression; p24 antigen, which is detectable in the serum of some patients, may show a rise at the same time and has been used as a marker of disease progression.

CD8 cytotoxic lymphocytes (CTL) capable of killing HIV-infected targets may have beneficial effects. This is suggested because viraemia declines at the time that CTL are first detected following infection and, in patients with stable disease, a high frequency of CTL is detectable in the peripheral blood. In addition, in individuals who have been regularly exposed to HIV whilst remaining seronegative and without detectable virus, HIV-specific CTL have been detected. As well as killing infected cells directly, CD8 lymphocytes may contribute to protection by producing several chemokines and CAF (CD8

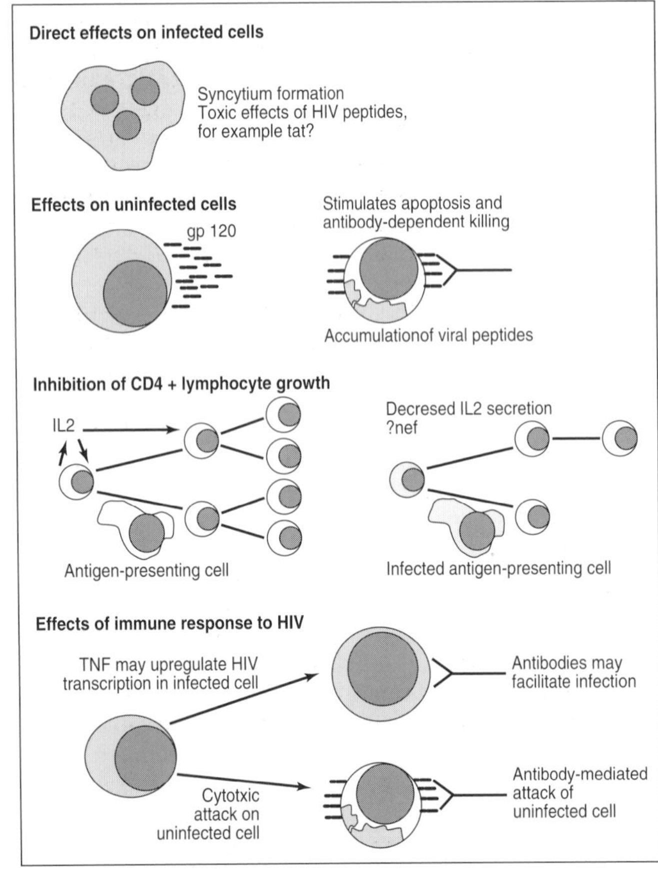

Mechanisms of CD4 lymphocyte loss in HIV infection.

Positive and negative effects of immune responses

- Antibody
  - Beneficial effects
    - Neutralising antibody (demonstated *in vitro* only) might prevent primary infection and destroy some infectious particles
    - Evidence for beneficial effect of passive transfer of antibody in man requires confirmation
  - Harmful effects
    - Antibody may also help the virus to enter cells with Fc receptors
    - Immune complexes may cause tissue damage, anaemia and neutropenia
- Cellular immune responses
  - Beneficial effects
    - A strong CD8 response is correlated with primary resistance in some individuals and with long-term survival
    - Cytotoxic T cells may delay the progress of disease by killing infected cells
    - They produce CD8 T cell antiviral factor (CAF) which inhibits viral replication and may be important in slowing disease progression
  - Harmful effects
    - They may kill uninfected cells which take up shed gp120
    - Abnormal cytokine secretion may cause immunopathology (perhaps including encephalopathy)

Protective mechanisms of CD8 T cells

	Cytotoxic	Non-cytotoxic
Mechanism	Death of infected cells	Inhibition of viral replication
Antigen specificity	Highly specific	Broad
Cell contact needed	Yes	Soluble factor (CAF) and possibly contact also
Genetic restriction	Yes	No
Induction by vaccination?	Yes	Not known

T cell antiviral factor), which strongly inhibit viral replication in CD4 cells. All this has led to the suggestion that CTL are an effective protective mechanism. However, because reverse transcription is an error-prone process, virus mutants arise, which evade the CTL response (escape mutants). These mutants may not only evade recognition themselves, but inhibit recognition of unmutated virus.

As well as contributing to protection, immune cells may mediate immunopathology. For example, several authors have shown that CTL can kill CD4 T cells, which have taken up free envelope glycoprotein shed from the surface of infected cells—a type of "innocent bystander lysis".

Monitoring HIV infection

Counting CD4 lymphocyte numbers (the "CD4 count") is an important part of monitoring HIV infection. A progressive downward trend in CD4 cells reflects disease progression and decreased life expectancy, even in the absence of symptoms. Epidemiological studies have firmly correlated distinct ranges of CD4 cell counts with risk of particular opportunist infections. Recent data show that monitoring either the absolute CD4 lymphocyte count or the ratio of CD4 to CD8 cells, the 4:8 ratio, are both equally good at monitoring progression in HIV infection. Serum levels of $\beta 2$-microglobulin and neopterin, which are molecules shed from activated lymphocytes, increase with progressive HIV infection and can be a useful adjunct to CD4 counts in monitoring.

Causes of CD4 lymphopenia

- HIV infection: seroconversion illness and during disease progression
- Acute viral infections*
- Tuberculosis*
- Sarcoidosis*
- Corticosteroid therapy
- Purine metabolism defects; ADA and PNP deficiency
- SLE

* Reduces CD4 counts when not associated with HIV and can further reduce levels in HIV infection

CD4 lymphocyte numbers have a diurnal variation and delays in the sample reaching the immunological laboratory (for example, when a sample is held overnight) also cause profound changes. Because CD4 lymphocyte counting is a lengthy process, most consistent results are obtained when samples are taken at a set time in the morning and sent straight to the lab. In the case of unavoidable hold-ups, samples should not be refrigerated.

CD4 counts should never be used as a substitute for an HIV test because low peripheral blood counts are seen in other conditions. The classic examples are sarcoidosis and tuberculosis (without HIV). Used inappropriately in these settings, a CD4 lymphocyte count may incorrectly suggest a diagnosis of HIV infection. CD4 counts may be low during seroconversion illness but usually recover initially during the asymptomatic phase. Hence there is a need to carry out several baseline CD4 counts if subsequent monitoring is to be useful.

Possibilities for immunotherapy

Attempts at immune reconstitution have been made using interleukin-2, interferons, thymic factors, or bone marrow transplantation. These have not been notably successful and remain

Immunotherapy for AIDS

Treatment	Outcome
α and γ interferons	Inconclusive
Interleukin-2	Inconclusive
Cyclosporin A	Not beneficial
Anti-HIV antiserum	Possible transient improvement
Bone marrow transplantation	Transient improvement in lymphocyte count and skin anergy

potentially harmful, since the very factors which activate T cells will also activate HIV replication. *In vivo* activation of CD4 cells is caused by stimulation with antigens in the form of micro-organisms or vaccines. This suggests that it is sensible to treat intercurrent infections promptly and provides a rationale for prophylactic chemotherapy for pheumocystis. In some studies, vaccination (for example with influenza vaccine) has been shown to be enough of an antigenic stimulus to increase HIV replication. Although not all studies show such HIV reactivation, this risk has to be considered along with the decreased efficacy of vaccines in HIV patients, particularly those with low CD4 counts or symptomatic disease. Live vaccines are always contraindicated.

The recent evidence of the powerful inhibitory effects of chemokines on HIV replication suggest that some lymphokines could provide therapeutic benefits and may lead to a resurgence of interest in immunotherapy.

Vaccine development

Strategies for vaccine development

- Should induce both neutralising antibody and CD8 T immunity
- Should contain both envelope and conserved portions of core antigens
- Induction of neutralising antibody requires native envelope while peptides are sufficient for CD8 T cell induction
- Peptides with novel adjuvants or live recombinant vectors containing HIV genes induce CD8 T cells
- DNA immunisation can generate both antibody and CD8 immunity

Immunisation against an organism whose target is an important component of the immune system presents particular difficulties. In addition, HIV has already been shown to be perhaps the most variable virus yet discovered, and HIV-2 differs greatly from all HIV-1 isolates. So far, efforts to immunise against the virus have concentrated on the use of cloned gp120, because all strains of virus so far tested use gp120 to bind to the CD4 molecule, implying that a part of the envelope is similar in all strains. In experimental animals gp120 does induce a neutralising antibody response to the virus but restricted to the immunising strain of virus (type-specific immunity). Furthermore, these neutralising sera do not provide reliable protection against virus challenge *in vivo* in animal experiments. The evidence, that when the antibody response to virus core antigen (p24) declines, the disease often progresses, suggests that an immune response to core antigens may be important. CTL are frequently specific for core antigens and the association of good prognosis and anticore antibody might therefore occur because there is concurrent protective T cell immunity. Some CTL are directed at relatively conserved sequences in core proteins and may be important in people infected with HIV but with no evidence of clinical progression. The identification of a variety of individuals exposed to HIV but with no evidence of infection, all exhibiting cellular immune responses to core proteins, reinforces the view that this type of response is important in protection. An effective vaccine might therefore contain components able to stimulate both neutralising antibody and strong CTL responses.

A key factor in generating immune responses is the way in which the antigens are presented to the immune system. For the generation of effective CTL responses, attenuated live viruses are effective and attenuated (nef-deleted) simian immunodeficiency virus (SIV) has been shown able to protect monkeys against challenge with virulent virus. While such a strategy is unlikely to be used in humans because of worries about the safety of such a virus, this is an encouraging result and HIV genes might be inserted by genetic engineering in a non-pathogenic virus "vector" such as vaccinia or adenovirus. In this way HIV antigens could be expressed in cells as in a normal infection, but without the possibility of HIV replicating and causing disease. Other means of delivery capable of inducing both antibody and cellular immunity, such as peptides or proteins in novel adjuvants, or naked DNA, are under active investigation.

Clearly neither antibody nor cell-mediated responses prevent the progression of disease in most patients but they may delay it. However, strong pre-existing humoral and cellular immunity induced by a vaccine might still be protective. Results of vaccination experiments in monkeys and the existence of individuals who appear to be resistant to HIV infection, provide grounds for cautious optimism with regard to the feasibility of producing HIV vaccines. Adequate testing of an HIV vaccine will be difficult in man, although the SIV model provides a model for vaccine development.

4 NATURAL HISTORY AND MANAGEMENT OF EARLY HIV INFECTION

Adrian Mindel, Melinda Tenant-Flowers

Summary of CDC 1992 classification system for HIV disease

Group I	Seroconversion illness
Group II	Asymptomatic infection
Group III	Persistent generalised lymphadenopathy
Group IV	Symptomatic infection
Group IVA	HIV wasting syndrome (AIDS) and constitutional disease
Group IVB	HIV encephalopathy (AIDS) and neurological disease
Group IVC1	Major opportunistic infections specified as AIDS defining
Group IVC2	Minor opportunistic infections
Group IVD	Cancers specified as AIDS defining
Group IVE	Other conditions

Infection with HIV causes a spectrum of clinical problems beginning at the time of seroconversion and terminating with AIDS and death. It is now recognised that it may take 10 years or more for AIDS to develop after seroconversion. The Centers for Disease Control (CDC) in the USA developed the most widely used classification for HIV disease based on the presence of clinical symptoms and signs, the presence of certain conditions and investigative findings, the availability of HIV screening, and the degree of immunosuppression as measured by the CD4 lymphocyte count. The infection is divided into four groups (see box).

Group I	Setoconversion
Group II	Asymptomatic phase
Group III	Persistent generalised lymphadenopathy
Group IV	Symptomatic infection

Summary of CDC 1993 classification system for HIV disease

	(1)	(2)	(3)
CD4 lymphocyte count $\times 10^6$/l	>500	200–499	<199
(A) Asymptomatic including Groups I, II and III	A1	A2	A3
(B) Symptomatic not A or C	B1	B2	B3
(C) AIDS-defining conditions	C1	C2	C3

Group IV is subdivided into several subgroups and some of these (groups IVA, B, C1 and D) are all AIDS-defining conditions.

In 1992 the CDC included all HIV-infected persons with CD4 lymphocyte counts of $< 200 \times 10^6$/l as fulfilling an AIDS-defining diagnosis. However, this additional classification is not widely used outside the USA.

A second classification also combines clinical and CD4 count information. Symptoms and clinical findings are graded in severity from A to C and CD4 counts as they fall from 1 to 3.

Group I Seroconversion illness

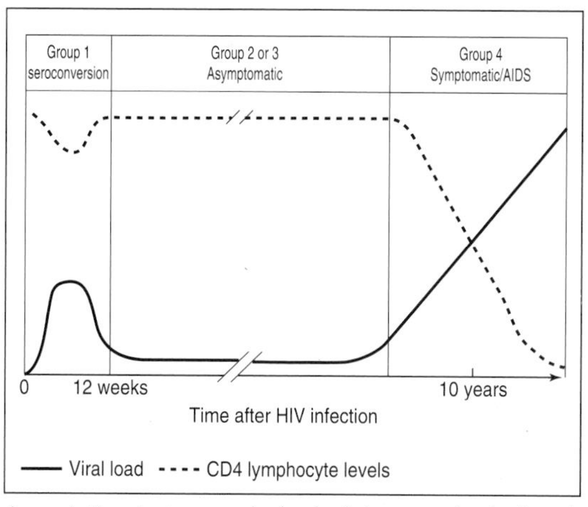

Association between virological, immunological and clinical events and time course of HIV infection.

This stage of HIV disease is also called the seroconversion illness or acute HIV infection. It represents the stage of infection after the acquisition of the virus when antibodies are developing as shown in the figure; 25–60% of people present with symptoms at the time of seroconversion. These can range from a mild, glandular fever-like illness to an encephalopathy. Common symptoms and signs are shown in the box. Severe symptoms are rare. The differential diagnosis of the mild seroconversion illness is protean and, without a high index of suspicion and a history indicating relevant risk behaviours or factors, the diagnosis may be missed. Investigations which may be useful in reaching a diagnosis are set out in the table.

Clinical manifestations of group I disease

- Glandular fever-like illness
- Fever, malaise, diarrhoea, neuralgia
- Arthralgia, sore throat, headaches
- Lymphadenopathy
- Macular papular rash
- Ulceration
  - oropharynx
  - anogenital area
- Neurological symptoms
  - meningitis
  - neuropathy
  - myelopathy
  - encephalopathy

Differential diagnosis of glandular fever-like illness

Condition	Test
Viral	
Infectious mononucleosis	Paul–Bunnell
Cytomegalovirus	Serology/culture
Rubella	Serology
Herpes simplex	HSV culture
Adenovirus	Serology
Hepatitis B/C	Serology
HIV	HIV Ab, Ag, PCR
Protozoal	
Toxoplasmosis	Serology
Bacterial	
Syphilis	Serology
Streptococcal pharyngitis	Bacterial culture
Brucellosis	Serology
Neoplastic	
Lymphoma or leukaemia	Full blood count/diff Lymph node biopsy Bone marrow

The appropriate diagnostic tests for seroconversion, which should be carried out on serial blood samples include tests for HIV antibodies and antigen. If these are negative and seroconversion is suspected, the definitive test is an HIV PCR, which is the most sensitive test for the detection and quantification of the virus. Some of these assays are not routine and the interpretation of investigation results during seroconversion is difficult, therefore close consultation with colleagues in the virology department is strongly advised. At the time of seroconversion there is sometimes a high rate of viral replication, leading to a transient rise in HIV viral load and concomitant immunosuppression due to a short-lived fall in the CD4 count. This may result in manifestations of HIV disease which are normally seen later in the infection, for example oral candida. This can lead to diagnostic confusion which can only be resolved by following the patient up for long enough to see the symptoms and signs resolve, HIV antibodies appear, the viral load fall, and the CD4 count rise. Treatment should be directed at alleviating any symptoms, and there is considerable interest in the possible use of antiretroviral agents at this time.

Group II Asymptomatic infection

After seroconversion, HIV antibodies continue to be detectable in the blood. The amount of virus detectable in blood and lymphoid tissues falls to very low levels and the rate of replication of HIV is slow although it does not stop. CD4 and CD8 lymphocyte counts are in the normal range and the infected person remains well. This phase may persist for as long as 10 years. The role of antiretroviral therapy during stage II infection is discussed in a later chapter.

Group III HIV and persistent lymphadenopathy

Persistent generalised lymphadenopathy may be a presenting feature of HIV infection in a person who is otherwise well. HIV-related lymphadenopathy persists for at least three months, in at least two extrainguinal sites and is not due to any other cause. The differential diagnosis of this lymphadenopathy is shown in the box above.

A lymph node biopsy in HIV disease is not recommended as a routine procedure as the findings are non-specific and the presence of lymphadenopathy due to HIV alone does not worsen the prognosis. The indications for a biopsy are the same in HIV and non-HIV-related conditions.

Indications for lymph node biopsy

- Constitutional symptoms
- Painful nodes
- Asymmetrical enlargement
- Sudden increase in size
- Hilar lymphadenopathy

Group IVA (Symptomatic HIV disease before the development of AIDS)

Late on in HIV infection, for reasons that we do not understand, viral replication increases and more CD4 and CD8 cells are destroyed. This results in a decline in immune competence and the appearance of symptoms, signs and infections at various sites. This overall decline in wellbeing proceeds at different rates for different individuals and is usually distressing. At this stage the CD4 count has usually dropped to around or below 200×10^6/l and prophylaxis for various infections and antiretroviral therapies should be discussed with the patient if these issues have not been raised before.

Constitutional symptoms

Constitutional symptoms in HIV infection

- Weight loss >10% baseline
- Fever lasting at least 1 month
- Diarrhoea lasting at least 1 month

The constitutional symptoms associated with HIV infection include malaise, fevers, night sweats, weight loss, and diarrhoea. These symptoms probably occur intermittently in many infected people and investigations should always be considered to discover possible treatable causes other than HIV. Many patients find these symptoms worrying and debilitating. The criteria for judging whether the symptoms are serious are set out in the box. It is worth noting that the combination of 10% weight loss from baseline and one other persistent symptom is an AIDS-defining condition. Once other causes have been excluded, treatment should be symptomatic using antipyretics and antidiarrhoeal agents. Antiretroviral therapy is often helpful and if all else fails steroids are sometimes useful.

Skin and mouth problems

Various minor skin problems occur in patients infected with HIV. Sometimes these are exacerbations of previous skin disease, but often they are new. The same conditions are often seen in persons not infected with HIV. However, in the presence of immunosuppression these common conditions may be more severe, persistent, and difficult to treat. Seborrhoeic dermatitis is frequently seen. It usually presents as a red scaly rash affecting the face and scalp, and sometimes the whole body. This condition usually responds well to 1% hydrocortisone and antifungal cream. Other common conditions include tinea cruris and pedis, candidiasis (particularly affecting the penis and perianal area), folliculitis, impetigo, and shingles. Recurrent perianal or genital herpes may become more troublesome, with recurrences lasting longer and occurring more frequently. Treatment with long-term aciclovir suppression is often required. Anogenital warts are common, difficult to treat and frequently recurrent, and high-grade cervical dysplasia is seen more often in HIV-infected women. The diagnosis of these skin conditions may be difficult; recurrences after adequate treatment often occur and expert help should be sought early.

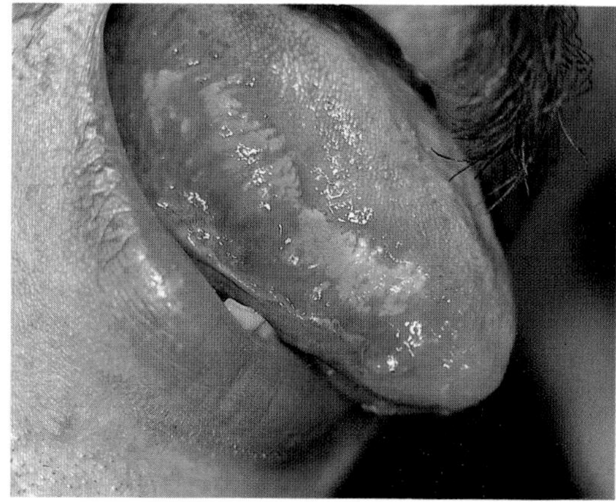

Hairy leukoplakia.

Mouth problems are also common and may cause considerable distress. Oral candida can be managed with topical or systemic antifungals such as ketoconazole or fluconazole. If dysphagia develops, oesophageal candidiasis should be suspected and investigated. Oral hairy leukoplakia can be differentiated from candida by its characteristic distribution along the lateral borders of the tongue and the fact that it cannot be scraped off. It contains Epstein–Barr virus. It is painless but unsightly and temporary remission can be obtained with aciclovir. Other oral conditions including dental abscesses, caries, gingivitis, and oral ulceration (herpetic or bacterial) may occur. Mouth

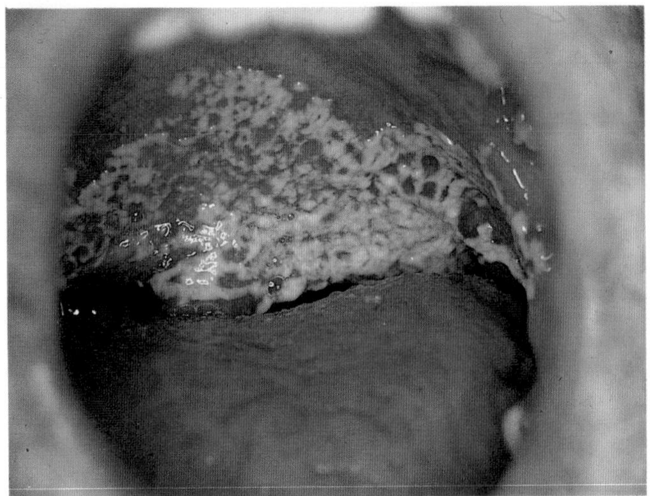
Oral candida.

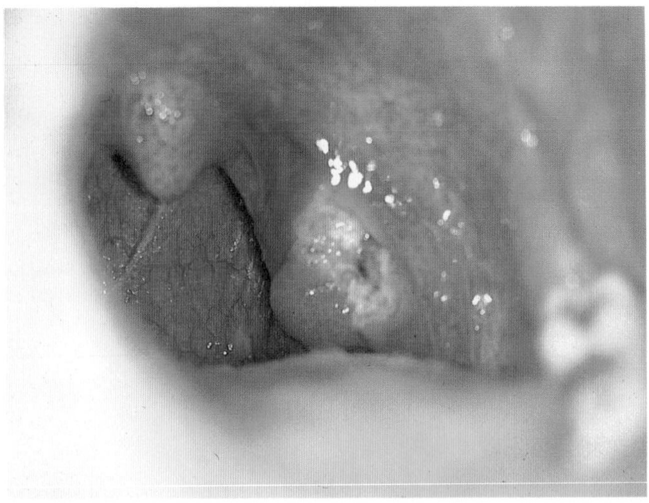
Mouth ulcer.

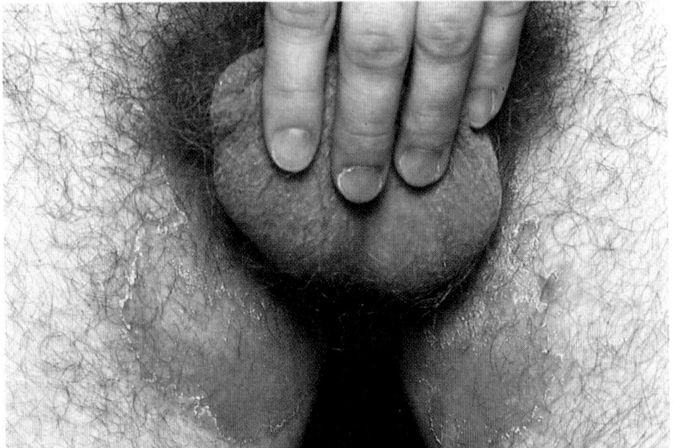
Tinea cruris.

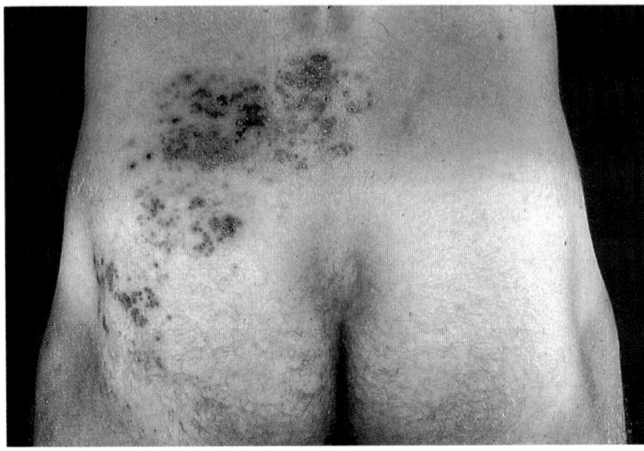
Varicella zoster.

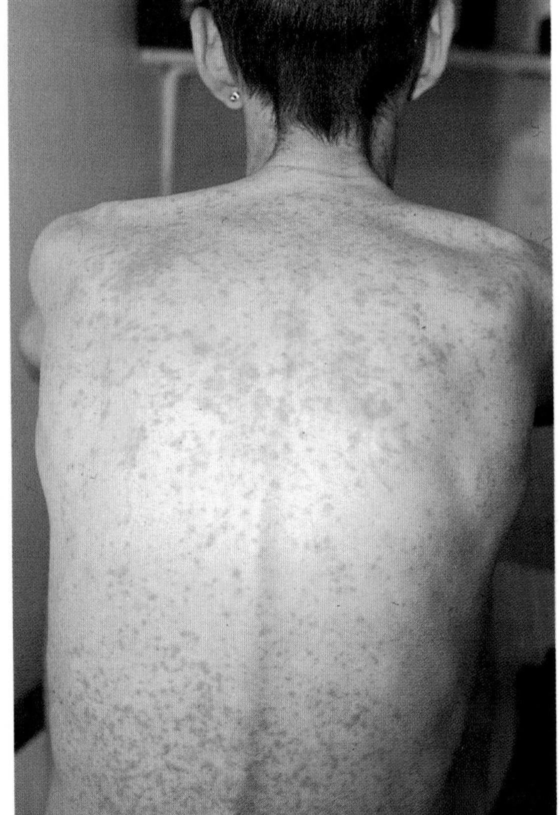
Extensive seborrhoeic dermatitis.

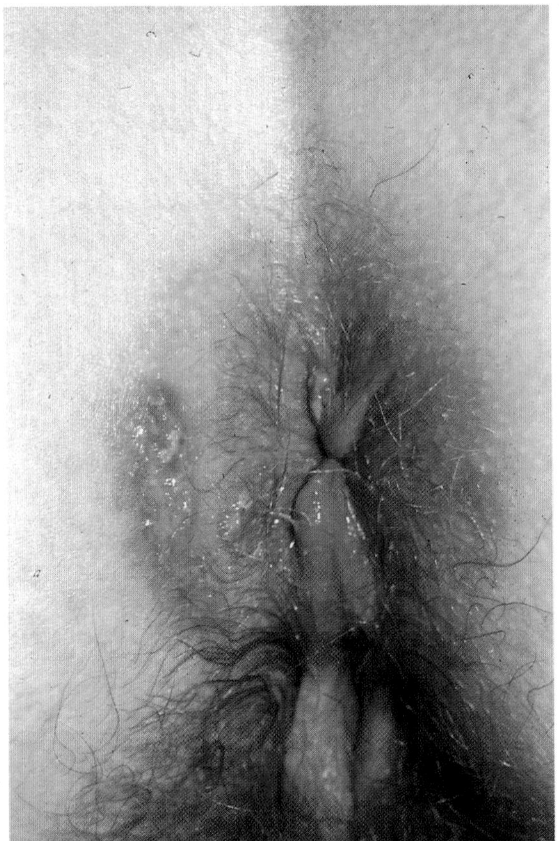
Perianal herpes.

Skin and mouth problems associated with HIV

Skin problems

- Miscellaneous
  - seborrhoeic dermatitis
- Fungal
  - tinea
    - cruris
    - pedis
    - other
  - candida
    - genital
    - perianal
    - other
  - pityriasis versicolor
- Bacterial
  - staphylococcal infection (impetigo)
  - acneform folliculitis
- Viral
  - herpes simplex (types 1 and 2)
    - oral
    - genital
    - perianal
    - other
  - varicella zoster
  - human papilloma virus
  - molluscum contagiosum
- Neoplastic
  - cervical dysplasia

Mouth problems

- Hairy oral leukoplakia
- Dental abscesses/caries
- Gingivitis
- Candidiasis
- Ulceration
  - bacterial
  - herpetic
  - aphthous

ulcers may be particularly difficult to treat and expert specialist assessment is recommended. Metronidazole, aciclovir, 0·2% chlorhexidine mouthwashes, and analgesic sprays may all be effective depending on the cause and, in extreme cases, thalidomide has been used. Maintenance of good oral hygiene and dental care is important. Oral Kaposi's sarcoma is often associated with disseminated lesions throughout the gastrointestinal tract.

HIV and haematological problems

Lymphopenia with depression of the CD4 cell subset is a hallmark of HIV disease. Mild to moderate neutropenia is commonly seen, but often does not adversely affect HIV-infected people. A normochromic, normocytic anaemia of unknown origin is also commonly seen. Severe anaemia should be investigated for other underlying causes. Thrombocytopenia is common in HIV disease and, only if persistent and $<20 \times 10^9/l$ warrants treatment with zidovudine, which is usually effective. Many therapies used to treat HIV or opportunistic infections and cancers may be toxic to bone marow.

Risk of progression and the value of prognostic markers

One of the hardest problems confronting the physician dealing with an asymptomatic patient with HIV infection is predicting how soon that patient will progress to AIDS. This issue is important, firstly, in terms of counselling and secondly, to decide which patients may benefit from antiretroviral treatment or prophylaxis to prevent opportunistic infections. These issues are discussed in Chapter 9. Patients who present with constitutional symptoms, persistent infections such as oral candida, and/or a CD4 count $<200 \times 10^6/l$ should be considered for prophylaxis against opportunistic infections and antiretroviral therapy.

A group of patients has recently been recognised who remain well with elevated CD4 and CD8 counts for a long time. These long-term survivors or non-progressors are under intensive study to define whether their prolonged wellbeing is due to viral, immunological, or other factors.

Variables associated with rapid disease progression include a symptomatic seroconversion illness, older age at diagnosis, and receipt of a large inoculum of virus, for example, via a contaminated transfusion from a donor with a high viral load. The effect of prophylaxis against opportunistic infections has been to delay the onset of AIDS and to change the pattern of disease represented by the first AIDS-defining illness. Antiretroviral treatment has independently been shown to increase survival before and after AIDS.

Markers of progression and treatment efficacy in HIV disease

- Immunological markers
  - CD4 cell counts
  - CD8 cell counts
  - CD4 percentages
  - Rate of change of serial CD4 counts
  - IgA
  - β2-microglobulin
  - Neopterin
- Virological markers
  - HIV p24 antigen
  - HIV viral load (PCR)

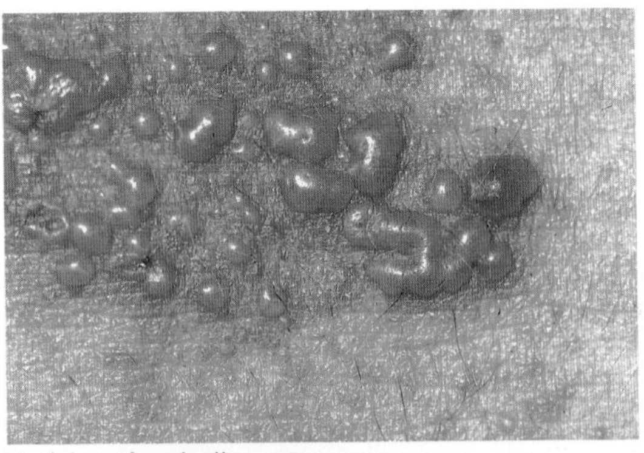
Vesicles of varicella zoster.

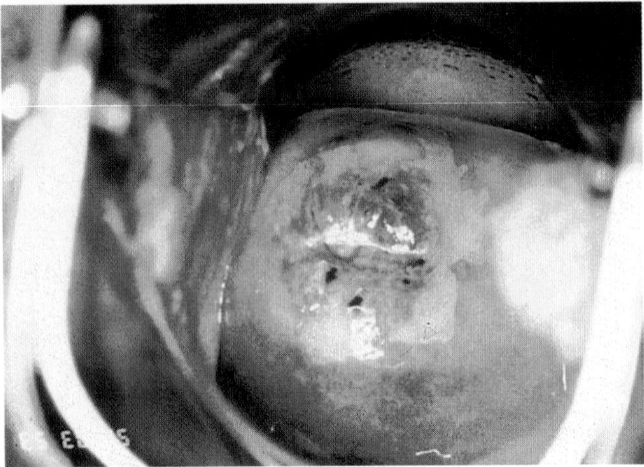
Cervical intraepithelial neoplasia.

Many laboratory markers are used as prognostic indicators, both to evaluate disease progression and the efficacy of treatment. The most widely used is the CD4 absolute lymphocyte count or percentage. The rate of decline of CD4 counts is also employed, particularly if this increases suddenly. However, CD4 counts should be interpreted with caution for several reasons. The count is subject to diurnal and seasonal variation and by intercurrent infection. Clinical decisions should not be based on the results of a single count but rather on the pattern over time. Other immunological markers that can be used in conjunction with CD4 counts are IgA, β2-microglobulin and neopterin levels which may all become elevated as HIV disease progresses.

Currently, there is much interest in measuring viral parameters and using these as markers of progression. This is because they are thought to be directly related to what is happening in HIV disease progression and treatment, whereas immunological markers may be depressed or elevated by other events. HIV p24 antigen has a limited application as it is only detectable in 50% of infected persons. Newer PCR-based techniques which directly measure amplified viral load or amplified signals from the virus (branched chain DNA) are under evaluation to establish their usefulness as markers of progression and response to therapy.

General management of HIV-infected people

One of the most important aspects of dealing with any HIV-infected person is confidentiality. Maintaining confidentiality might be complicated: for example, the patient's family or friends may not know his or her diagnosis or sexual orientation; people at work (or school) may seek medical information (especially if the patient is having time off work); or the patient may fear that information could inadvertently be given to third parties. Special precautions may be required, firstly, to reassure the patient that confidentiality is protected and, secondly, to limit any unwarranted dissemination of confidential information.

The routine medical management of these patients is usually straightforward. Patients should be seen regularly, for example every two to three months. At each visit the patient's weight should be recorded and special attention given to mouth or skin problems. If necessary the patient should be referred to the appropriate specialist. Repeating a full blood count and measuring the CD4 count every three to six months is often helpful. Patients should be advised to reattend if they develop symptoms suggesting opportunistic infections or cancers, for example, shortness of breath, cough, pain or difficulty swallowing, diarrhoea, weight loss, fevers, headaches, fitting, altered consciousness, or purple spots on the skin.

General management of the HIV infected person

- Protect confidentiality
- Medical issues
- Psychological support (patient, family, and friends)
- Avoidance of transmission
- Other issues (dental treatment, insurance, work or school, etc.)

Patients should also be advised about reducing the risk of transmission. Psychological and emotional support of the patient, family, and friends are a vital aspect of management (see chapter 13), and advice concerning safer sex, safer needle use, pregnancy, breastfeeding, and children should also be provided. The physician may also be asked to advise about dental treatment, insurance, and work. Patients should be advised to tell their dentists about their infection, and it may sometimes be necessary to refer them to a dental unit with an interest in HIV-related problems. Infected people will often have considerable difficulty in obtaining life insurance as most insurance companies ask specific questions about the infection and either refuse insurance or charge very high premiums. Finally, patients should be told that being positive is no barrier to employment provided there is no chance of their body fluids entering another person or of them transmitting an opportunistic infection, such as tuberculosis by coughing. Because of widespread misconceptions about infectivity which are still prevalent, information about the patient's condition should not be divulged to employers without their consent.

5 TUMOURS

Paul Rogers, Margaret Spittle

Risk of malignancies in HIV-positive patients

Malignancy	Relative risk compared to HIV-negative population	Viral co-factor
Kaposi's sarcoma	716–972	KSHV (HHV8)
NHL	71–141	EBV
Primary CNS lymphoma (PCNSL)	~100	EBV
Cervical cancer	?	HPV
Hodgkin's disease	5–9	EBV
Anal cancer	3·5–5	HPV
Testicular germ cell tumours	3	?

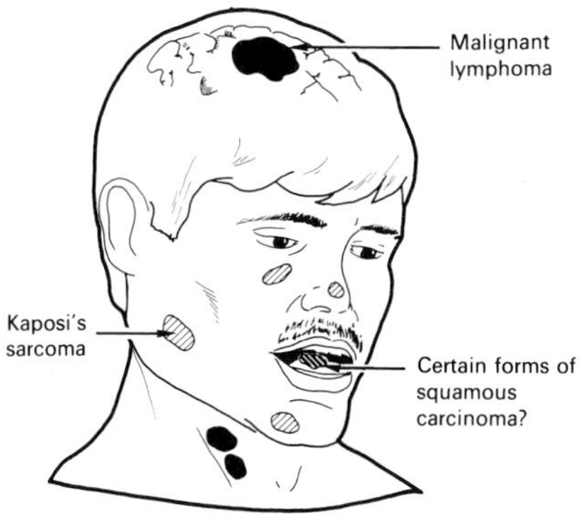

AIDS-related tumour sites. (Courtesy of the late Dr Neil Smith.)

There are currently four malignancies recognised by the US Centers for Disease Control (US-CDC) which define the onset of AIDS in HIV-positive patients. These are Kaposi's sarcoma, non-Hodgkin's lymphoma, primary CNS lymphoma and, since 1993, cervical cancer. Epidemiological studies have shown that HIV-positive patients are also at increased risk of other malignancies including Hodgkin's disease, anal cancer, and testicular germ cell tumours.

It appears that viral co-factors play an important role in HIV-related malignancies. By causing immunodeficiency HIV allows increased expression of certain oncogenic viruses. The causal relationships between the Epstein–Barr virus (EBV) and lymphomas and the human papilloma virus (HPV) and squamous carcinomas of the cervix and anus is well documented. A sexually transmitted agent is thought to be responsible for HIV-related Kaposi's sarcoma. The Kaposi's sarcoma herpes virus (KSHV), also known as the human herpes virus 8 (HHV8), has been identified in Kaposi's sarcomas and body fluids, including semen, from homosexual men. The precise role of KSHV is not yet fully understood.

Kaposi's sarcoma

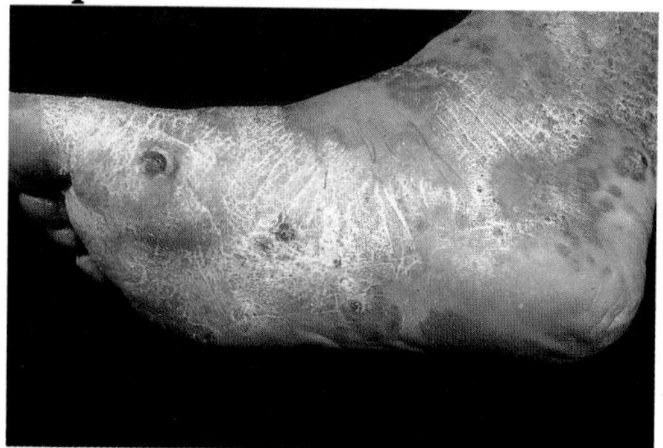

Classic Kaposi's sarcoma on the foot of an elderly man.

Clinical groups of patients with Kaposi's sarcoma (KS)

(1) "Classic" KS: elderly, predominantly male, Jewish or Eastern European
(2) "Endemic" or African KS (various types)
(3) Immunosuppression-related KS (patients with transplants)
(4) "Epidemic" or AIDS-related KS

In the wake of the HIV epidemic, Kaposi's sarcoma (KS) is seen commonly in AIDS patients, and the aetiology and pathogenesis are becoming clearer. There are four clinical groups of patients with KS.

The "classic" form is seen mainly on the legs of elderly Jewish or Eastern European patients. In this group it is 10–15 times more common in men than women. The course of the disease is slow and many patients die in old age of unrelated conditions.

"Endemic KS" has been present in sub-Saharan Africa for many years. In addition to a form resembling the classic KS, there is an aggressive variety which affects young adults and has many features in common with AIDS-related KS. In infants, KS usually presents with lymphadenopathy. In the equatorial "HIV belt" the AIDS-related variety is now also seen. African HIV-related KS occurs in both men and women, reflecting the heterosexual transmission of HIV.

Immunosuppression-related KS occurs in patients iatrogenically immunocompromised, for example, following renal transplants and in autoimmune diseases such as rheumatoid arthritis. Men and women are equally affected. The tumour may regress after reduction or cessation of immunosuppressive therapy.

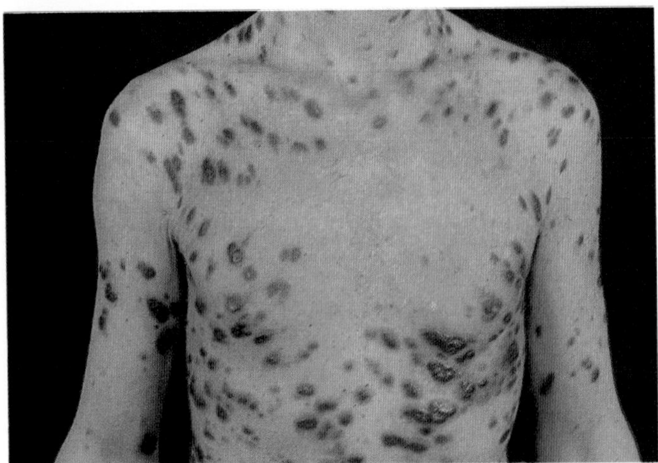

Widespread nodular cutaneous Kaposis' sarcoma.

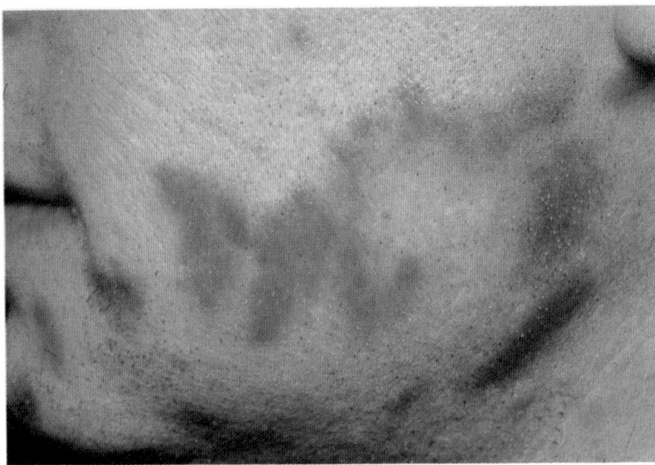

Early facial Kaposi's sarcoma.

"Epidemic" or AIDS-related KS is the commonest form seen in Britain. It predominantly affects young homosexual HIV-positive males rather than the other groups with HIV. It affects 3–4% of patients who have acquired HIV through intravenous drug usage or blood transfusions and 1% of HIV-positive haemophiliacs. KS was the AIDS-defining diagnosis in 30% of patients but now it accounts for 15%. The cause of the reduction is uncertain but presumably reflects the changing practices of homosexuals. More recently a viral agent that could be transmitted sexually has been isolated (see below). Changing sexual practices may be associated with reduced incidence of KS in this group. AIDS-related KS has a wide spectrum of behaviour but it usually becomes increasingly aggressive. The cutaneous form is a stigma which alarms HIV patients, particularly when lesions affect the face. Development of KS commonly precedes opportunistic infections. With the improvements in treating opportunistic infections, KS now accounts for the death of one in four HIV-positive homosexuals due to visceral, especially pulmonary, involvement.

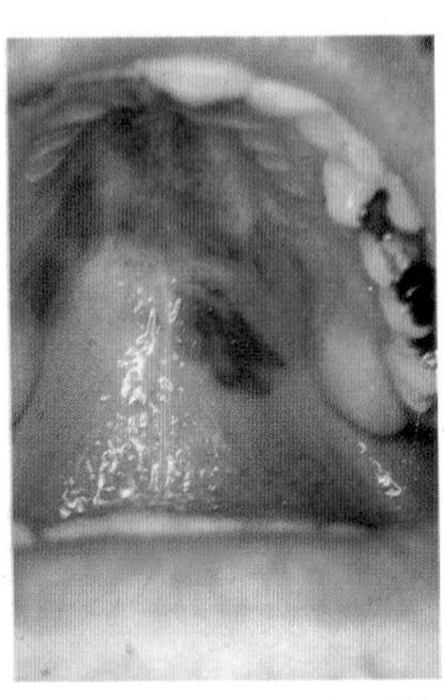

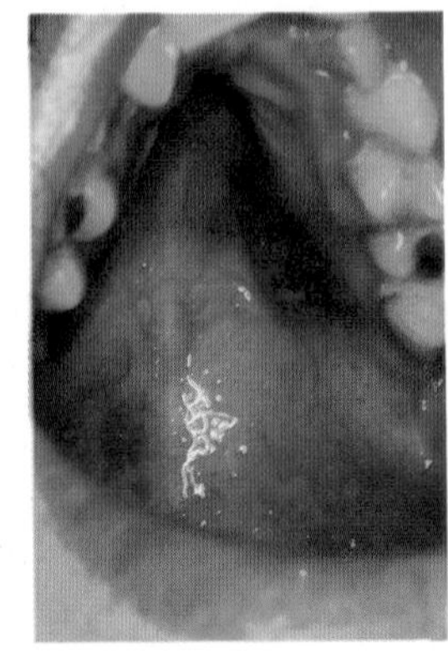

Mucocutaneous palatal Kaposi's sarcoma.

Clinical features and investigations

AIDS-related KS is usually multifocal and often progresses rapidly. Cutaneous lesions begin as small flat dusky red or violet areas of skin discolouration, progressing over weeks or months to raised painless firm nodules and plaques. Common sites involved include the legs, trunk, arms, face, hard palate, tip of nose, and penis. Tissue oedema is commonly present when KS affects the face, genitalia, and lower legs.

Mucocutaneous KS strongly predicts that the patient will also have, or will develop, visceral involvement. The lungs and gastrointestinal systems are most commonly involved. Pulmonary KS accounts for one third of respiratory episodes in patients with cutaneous KS. The untreated median survival of patients with pulmonary KS is 6 months (see chapter 6).

Gastrointestinal KS is often asymptomatic but may cause a protein-losing enteropathy, diarrhoea, bleeding, or pain. Diagnosis is by endoscopy (see chapter 7).

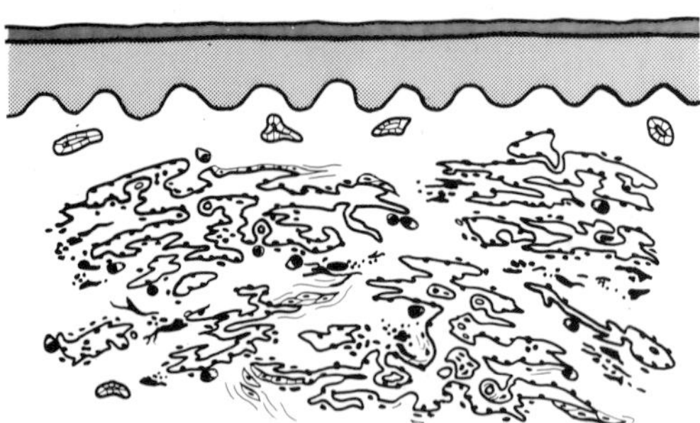

Lymphangioma-like Kaposi's sarcoma. (Courtesy of the late Dr Neil Smith.)

Pathogenesis

KS is a multifocal, multiorgan neoplasm consisting of aberrant vascular structures lined by abnormal endothelial cells and extravasated erythrocytes with a mononuclear cell infiltrate (predominantly plasma cells). The malignant cell is the spindle cell, a mesenchymal cell lying between the vessels. The tumour immunocytochemistry stains are positive for factor VIII and smooth muscle-specific α actin. The histopathological appearances of early cutaneous lesions are subtle and can easily be missed. Elongated and irregular spaces appear in the dermis. The patch stage (flat) may be composed of areas of these anastomosing spaces with a jagged outline and very little evidence of the tumour cell. This is the "lymphangioma-like" type of KS. The more advanced plaque and tumour stage lesions are more easily recognisable.

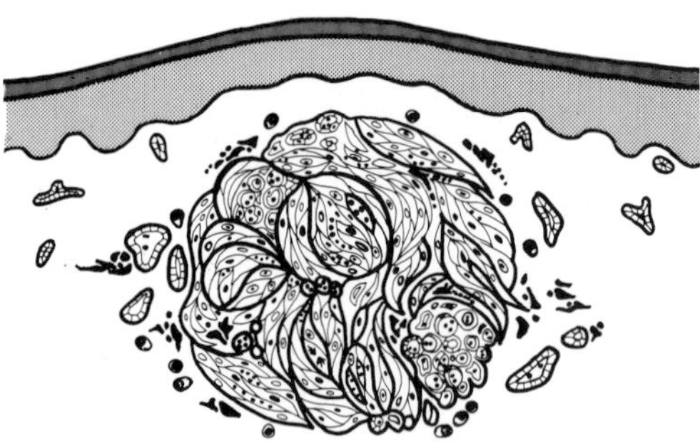

Classical nodular Kaposi's sarcoma. (Courtesy of the late Dr Neil Smith.)

Recent advances suggest that a herpes virus may be the cause of KS. DNA sequences from the human herpes virus 8 (HHV8), or "Kaposi's sarcoma herpes virus" (KSHV), have been identified in KS lesions, blood, semen, bronchial washings, and saliva of HIV-positive men. Furthermore, the DNA has been identified in non-HIV-related KS. This hypothesis fits in with epidemiological data suggesting that KS is caused by a sexually transmitted agent.

Another advance in understanding the pathogenesis of KS is the identification of cytokines which promote the growth of KS cells *in vitro*, for example interleukin 6 (IL-6), tumour necrosis factor (TNF), basic fibroblast growth factor (bFGF), vascular endothelial growth factor (VEGF), platelet-derived growth factor (PDGF), Oncostatin M, and granulocyte colony-stimulating factor (GCSF).

Treatment

The aim of treatment is to prolong life and maintain its quality. Both AIDS and AIDS-related KS are ultimately fatal diseases currently without a cure. The greatest risk of death is from opportunistic infections. However, with improved prophylaxis and treatment of opportunistic infections, more patients are developing life-threatening KS. Treatment should be tailored to the individual's disease. Local treatment for cosmesis is extremely important with this stigmatising condition. Local therapy ranges from camouflage with commercially available cosmetics, intralesional therapy with vinblastine or interferon, to radiotherapy.

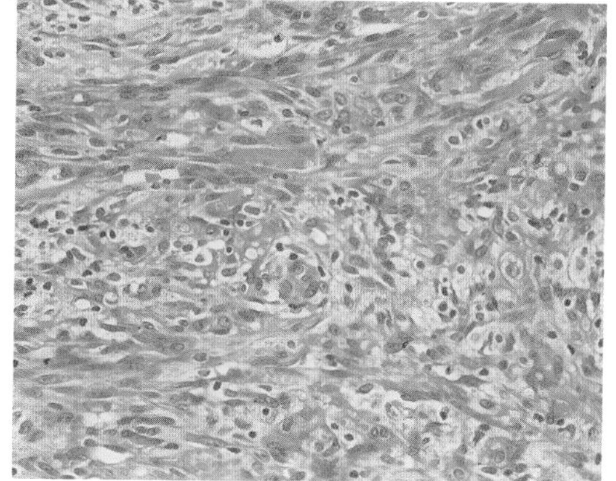

Spindle cell proliferation of nodular Kaposi's sarcoma.

Irradiation with a single fraction of 8 Gy using 100 kV photons has a 70% response rate, especially if the KS is early and has little haemosiderin staining. This dose may be repeated if further regression is required or relapse occurs. A unique mucosal sensitivity to radiotherapy may occur and fractionated regimens are required, for example, 15 Gy in 10 fractions using megavoltage photons. Alternatively, palatal brachytherapy is an effective and relatively non-toxic technique. Radiotherapy is particularly effective in controlling bleeding lesions.

Systemic treatment (immunotherapy or chemotherapy) is required when the pace of the disease is too great for local treatment, or when visceral involvement has become symptomatic. When the CD4 count is above $200 \times 10^6/l$, immunotherapy with interferon α has the advantage that it is unlikely to cause neutropenia. It has also been suggested that some patients experience less overwhelming opportunistic infections during treatment. The patient commences 3 MU *nocte*, subcutaneously on alternate days. Provided the side effects of fevers, shivering, and malaise are tolerated, dose escalation to 10–30 MU gives the best results.

KS may appear when the CD4 count has fallen to $50–100 \times 10^6/l$. These patients are already seriously immunocompromised and chemotherapy may lower the CD4 count even further. Bleomycin and vincristine have the least effect on the bone marrow and these two drugs have been the gold standard of chemotherapy for a long time, giving responses in 50–60% of patients. The tumour flattens, fades and, in some instances, totally regresses. The side effects although not common, can be unpleasant: bleomycin may cause a dose-related interstitial pneumonia or pulmonary fibrosis whilst vincristine may cause a peripheral neuropathy. In the United States, doxorubicin is added but this causes alopecia which is also a stigmatising condition which patients want to avoid. Other serious side effects of doxorubicin include bone marrow depression and cardiotoxicity when the total dose exceeds 450–550 mg/m^2. These problems may be minimised by "packaging" the drug in liposomes—spheres of phospholipid bilayers which are selectively distributed in the tumours where the drug is deposited when the liposome breaks down. Some liposomes include an outer layer of polyethylene glycol which binds its own weight in water and therefore becomes invisible to the body's immune system. Preventing uptake in the bone marrow may reduce bone marrow toxicity. Response rates of up to 80–90% are seen, including prevention of new lesion formation as well.

New drugs currently under invesitgation in drug-resistant disease include the taxols, retinoic acid, β-HCG and anti-angiogenic agents such as thalidomide.

Non-Hodgkin's lymphoma

B symptoms

- Loss of weight (>10% body weight in 6 months)
- Fevers >38°C
- Night sweats

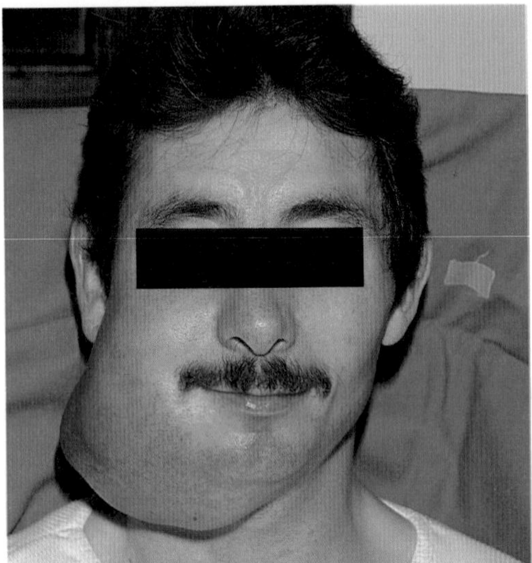

Aggressive presentation of nodal lymphoma.

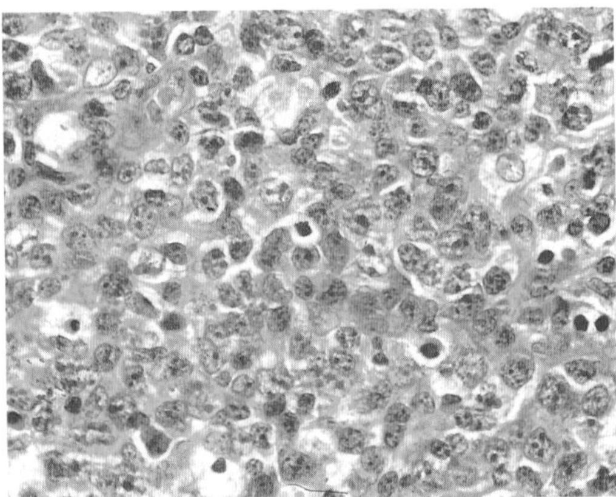

High grade (lymphoblastic) malignant lymphoma.

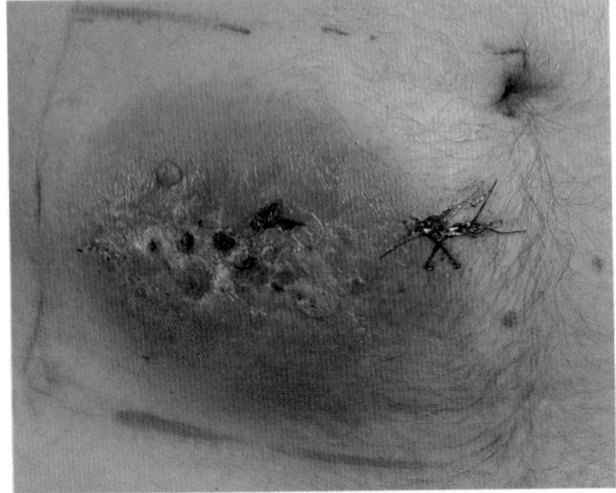

Presenting mass of extranodal lymphoma in abdominal wall.

Poor prognostic risk factors

- Poor performance status
  - confined to bed during waking hours
  - at best, capable of self care only
- Previous AIDS-defining diagnosis
- CD4 count $<100 \times 10^6$/l

Non-Hodgkin's lymphoma (NHL) is the second most frequent AIDS-defining malignancy. Unlike Kaposi's sarcoma, NHL is seen in all risk groups with AIDS. NHL is seen more frequently in Italy, where the main risk factor is intravenous drug usage, than in England. No causal factor for this has been found. AIDS-related NHL accounts for 3% of all cases of NHL and occurs in 3% of all risk groups. It is seen over 100 times more frequently than in the HIV-negative population. About half those developing AIDS-related NHL already have an AIDS-defining diagnosis. Patients with severe immunodeficiency who survive for up to three years with antiviral therapy have a higher probability of developing NHL. The proportion developing NHL is predicted to increase because of the longer survival of patients with HIV infection.

Pathogenesis

A co-virus seems to be responsible for this HIV-related malignancy. The Epstein–Barr virus (EBV) is closely linked with the development of lymphoma in AIDS. EBV proteins are demonstrable in virtually all primary CNS lymphomas and 50% of nodal and other extranodal sites.

Most cases are high grade B cell lymphomas. In the Kiel classification the most common subtypes are immunoblastic, centroblastic, lymphoblastic, or Burkitt-like lymphoma.

Clinical features and investigations

The presentation is usually in 30–40-year-olds and the clinical features are varied. The features which differentiate AIDS-related NHL from that in immunocompetent patients include a higher frequency of B-symptoms, more extranodal disease and a more advanced stage of presentation.

A diagnostic biopsy is essential because of the frequent atypical presentation and the many alternative conditions producing lymphadenopathy in these patients. Staging investigations include chest X-ray, CT scan, and bone marrow biopsy. Unlike NHL in HIV-negative patients, the chance of CNS involvement is high and therefore a lumbar puncture should also be performed (after imaging the brain with CT or MRI to exclude cerebral masses which may present a risk of coning). Prognostic information is also obtained from full blood count, erythrocyte sedimentation rate and lactate dehydrogenase. The renal function must be assessed with U & Es prior to treatment which can cause acute renal failure due to tumour lysis syndrome and hyperuricaemia.

The median survival from systemic AIDS-related NHL is six months. Half die from opportunistic infection and half from the lymphoma. Primary CNS lymphoma has a much poorer prognosis.

Treatment

Localised disease can be treated with radiotherapy which has the advantage of not further compromising the bone marrow. More advanced disease requires chemotherapy. The ability to tolerate cytotoxic drugs which cause bone marrow depression is already low but there are three further important prognostic factors.

Low risk patients have no risk factors, "medium risk" have one factor whilst "high risk" have more than one factor. A European multinational trial is currently evaluating various regimens with differing degrees of bone marrow toxicity.

The standard treatment in low risk patients is CHOP (cyclophosphamide, doxorubicin, vincristine, and prednisolone). Various more intensive regimens have been tried such as M-BACOD (methotrexate, bleomycin, doxorubicin, cyclophosphamide, vincristine, and dexamethasone). Prophylactic intrathecal methotrexate or cytarabine in association with the less intensive regimens have comparable results but produce less opportunistic infections. Zidovudine (AZT) may be used as maintenance therapy.

Primary CNS lymphoma

Primary CNS lymphoma (PCNSL) affects 2–6% of HIV-positive individuals. This is much higher than the general population in which it accounts for 0·5–1·2% of all intracranial neoplasms. It is associated with other immunodeficiency states, both acquired and iatrogenic. In 1981 the US-CDC recognised this as an AIDS-definition criteria. Since then this proportion has remained surprisingly constant. It usually occurs in advanced AIDS when the CD4 counts are low. The patients often have other serious opportunistic infections such as cytomegalovirus, *Mycobacterium avium intracellulare* or toxoplasmosis.

Pathology

The histology is similar to that of systemic AIDS-related NHL except that almost all cases are also related to Epstein–Barr virus.

Clinical features and investigation

See chapter 8.

Treatment

Radiotherapy to the whole brain, with steroids, or intrathecal chemotherapy produces a median survival of 12–18 months in good performance patients who complete therapy. There have been no prospective trials to ascertain the optimum dose or fractionation. Without treatment the median survival is only 1·8 to 3·3 months. Most patients have a complete response to radiotherapy but relapse quickly in distant sites within the CNS.

Other tumours

Cervical cancer was made an AIDS-defining diagnosis by the US-CDC in 1993 but this is now debatable. There is little to confirm that this is no more than an epiphenomenon, that is HIV and cervical cancer are seen together because they are both related to sexual behaviour. The human papilloma virus (HPV) is a co-factor in this malignancy in both HIV-positive and -negative women. HPV is necessary, but not sufficient, for the progression of cervical intraepithelial neoplasia (CIN) to cervical cancer. Other factors are required, including immunosuppression and smoking.

Hodgkin's disease has an increased incidence of five to nine times in HIV-positive patients compared with the general population. There is a higher frequency of the mixed cellularity and lymphocyte-depleted subtypes with more advanced stage at presentation. Treatment with standard chemotherapy regimens such as ABVD (doxorubicin, bleomycin, vinblastine, and dacarbazine) are immunosuppressive in their own right and prophylaxis against OIs is important. Zidovudine also reduces the incidence of OIs.

Anal cancer is also related to HPV and HIV infection. It not only has an increased incidence in gay men practising anoreceptive intercourse but it is approximately five times more common in HIV-positive homosexuals than their HIV-negative counterparts.

Testicular germ cell tumours are three times more common in homosexual HIV-positive men. There is a much higher incidence of seminoma than teratoma. The reason for this is unclear.

6 AIDS AND THE LUNG

Rob Miller

HIV-associated respiratory disease

- *Pneumocystis carinii* pneumonia
- Bacterial infections
- Kaposi's sarcoma
- Tuberculosis
- *Mycobacterium avium intracellulare*
- Fungal pneumonia
- Lymphoma
- Lymphoid interstitial pneumonitis
- Non-specific interstitial pneumonitis

The lungs are commonly affected in patients infected with HIV, with over 60% of patients having at least one respiratory episode during the course of their disease. Over recent years there have been several changes in the pattern of lung disease seen in those infected with HIV. These changes may be accounted for by several factors including better education of patients, resulting in earlier presentation with clinical complications, and earlier detection of disease in out patients together with better treatment of opportunistic infection, and the increasing use of both primary and secondary prophylaxis for *Pneumocystis carinii* pneumonia.

Investigations

Investigation of respiratory disease

Non-invasive tests

Chest radiograph
Arterial blood gases or oximetry
Pulmonary function tests
Radionuclide scanning
Gallium 67 citrate
Technetium DTPA

Invasive tests

Induced sputum
Fibreoptic bronchoscopy and bronchoalveolar lavage with or without transbronchial biopsy
Open lung biopsy

Symptoms of cough and dyspnoea with or without fever and sweats identify the presence of respiratory disease in HIV-positive patients, but these are non-specific and symptomatic patients should be investigated.

Non-invasive investigations

These tests should ideally allow a specific diagnosis to be made and a therapeutic response monitored by a quick cheap, and universally available, method. Unfortunately, none of these tests fulfils the criteria but they do help to:

- determine the presence or absence of pulmonary disease;
- assess disease severity;
- determine if an invasive test is indicated to make an aetiological diagnosis.

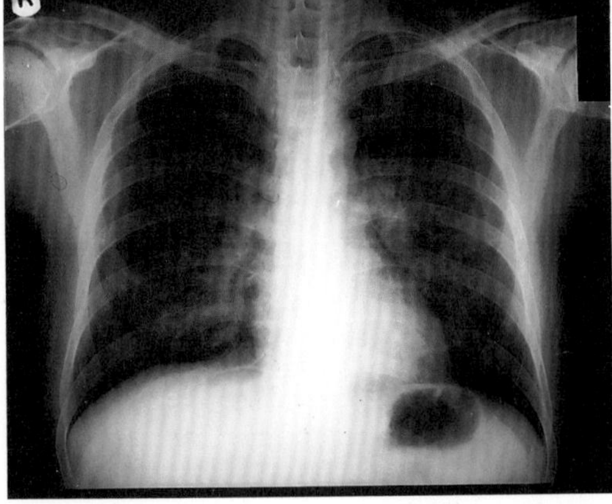

Chest radiograph of patient with early pneumocystis pneumonia.

Chest radiology—Chest radiography may be normal in HIV-positive patients with respiratory disease caused by *P. carinii* pneumonia and *Mycobacterium avium intracellulare* infection. The most common abnormality seen in patients with pneumocystis pneumonia is bilateral perihilar haze which may be very subtle and easy to miss. More severely unwell patients may have more diffuse interstitial shadowing which may progress to severe consolidation with "white out" throughout both lung fields, with sparing of the apices and costophrenic angles. These radiographic appearances are non-specific and may also be seen in pyogenic bacterial, mycobacterial, and fungal infection, and also in Kaposi's sarcoma and lymphoid interstitial pneumonitis. Between 5% and 10% of patients with pneumocystis pneumonia have atypical chest radiographs showing cystic changes, upper lobe infiltrates mimicking tuberculosis, hilar or mediastinal lymphadenopathy, or focal consolidation. The chest radiograph in pneumocystis pneumonia may deteriorate very rapidly from being normal to showing severe abnormality in just a few days. In contrast, radiographic recovery can be slow. Nodular shadowing, adenopathy, and pleural effusions on the chest radiograph suggest *M. tuberculosis*, Kaposi's sarcoma, or lymphoma.

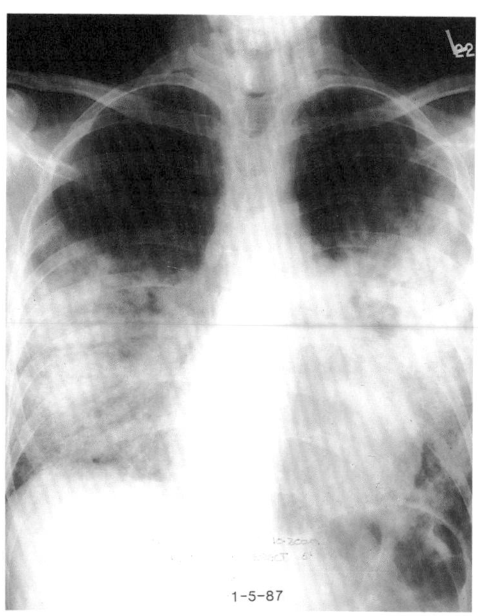

Chest radiograph of patient with severe pneumocystis pneumonia.

Arterial blood gases and oximetry—Hypoxaemia and a widened alveolar–arterial oxygen gradient are very sensitive for the diagnosis of pneumocystis pneumonia but may also occur in other conditions. Excercise-induced arterial desaturation detected by oximetry is also sensitive for the diagnosis of pneumocystis pneumonia; desaturation may also occur rarely in cytomegalovirus pneumonitis but is unusual in other respiratory conditions.

Pulmonary function tests—The single breath carbon monoxide transfer factor (TLCO), transfer coefficient (KCO), total lung capacity (TLC), and vital capacity (VC) may all be reduced in patients with pneumocystis pneumonia. Reductions in TLCO to ≤70% of predicted normal occur in HIV-positive patients with pneumocystis and other respiratory disease, including Kaposi's sarcoma and bacterial infections, so this finding is not specific.

Radionuclide scans—

(*a*) *Gallium 67 citrate*: This detects pulmonary inflammation. Diffuse intrapulmonary accumulation occurs in pneumocystis pneumonia but a similar pattern may also be seen in bacterial, fungal, and mycobacterial infection, and also in HIV-positive injecting drug users without overt respiratory disease. Gallium 67 citrate does not accumulate in pulmonary Kaposi's sarcoma lesions and so is useful in differentiating this diagnosis from infection. Focal intrapulmonary accumulation of gallium occurs most frequently in patients with mycobacterial and bacterial infection but is occasionally also seen in pneumocystis pneumonia.

(*b*) *Technetium-labelled diethylene triamene penta-acetic acid (Tc-DTPA)*: Clearance of aerosolised Tc-DTPA from the lungs is a measure of pulmonary epithelial permeability or "leakiness". Tc-DTPA clearance is very rapid in patients with pneumocystis pneumonia and the clearance curve is biphasic. This allows distinction to be made from HIV-positive smokers who also have an increased rate of Tc-DTPA clearance.

Invasive tests

These allow an aetiological diagnosis to be made.

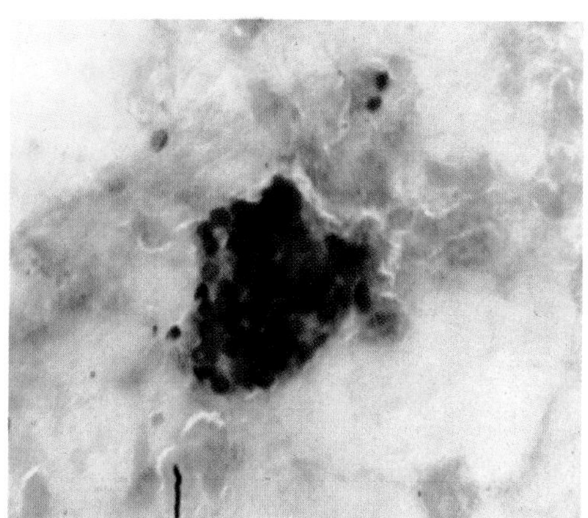

Cytology preparation of induced sputum showing many cysts of *Pneumocystis carinii* (Grocott's methenamine silver stain). (Courtesy of Dr Gabrijela Kocjan.)

Sputum induced by hypertonic saline—The patient inhales 20–30 ml of 2·7% (3N) saline through an ultrasonic nebuliser. Saline deposits in the peripheral airways and alveoli, causing irritation and inducing bronchial secretion. Fluid is also drawn into the airways from the interstitium, loosening inflammatory exudate and casts from alveoli. These are mobilised by the mucociliary staircase and move centrally where they are coughed out by the patient. Careful preparation of the patient is needed including an overnight starve and rigorous cleaning of the mouth to remove oral debris so that the sputum sample is not contaminated (food debris and squames take up stain and make analysis difficult). Purulent samples of sputum suggest a bacterial cause. *P. carinii* infection is usually found in clear "saliva-like" samples that become viscid on cooling to room temperature. Fungal infection and mycobacterial infection may also be diagnosed by this technique. Many centres do not carry out sputum induction because of the need for special equipment and the low yield when the technique is compared with fibreoptic bronchoscopy, both for the diagnosis of pneumocystis pneumonia and other pathogens. Some patients find sputum induction unpleasant and become nauseated or dyspnoeic. Arterial desaturation may also occur during the procedure.

Fibreoptic bronchosocpy—Bronchoscopy allows inspection of the bronchi to be carried out and lesions of Kaposi's sarcoma may be identified. Bronchoalveolar lavage is routinely carried out from the right middle lobe or from the area of maximum abnormality seen on the chest radiograph. Transbronchial biopsies are now rarely done as they add little to the diagnostic yield for *P. carinii* and other diagnoses, and the technique is associated with adverse effects including haemorrhage and pneumothorax. If transbronchial biopsy is not performed a diagnosis of non-specific or lymphoid interstitial pneumonitis might be missed.

Open lung biopsy

If fibreoptic bronchoscopy and lavage fail to identify diagnosis

or

where patient with bronchoscopic diagnosis deteriorates despite specific treatment

Open lung biopsy—It is rarely necessary to carry out open lung biopsy because of the high yield from bronchoalveolar lavage. This investigation may be necessary if fibreoptic bronchoscopy and lavage fail to identify diagnosis or in cases where a patient with a bronchoscopic diagnosis deteriorates despite specific treatment. The presenting clinical features and treatment of the common pulmonary manifestations of HIV disease are described below.

Pneumocystis carinii pneumonia

Pneumocystis carinni pneumonia remains the commonest pulmonary infection in AIDS, accounting for about half of all episodes. Patients complain of a non-productive cough and increasing dyspnoea (over two to three weeks or more); they may also have fever and sweats. The chest radiograph may be normal or show interstitial infiltrates: in severe pneumonia there may be a widespread alveolar consolidation.

Grading of severity of *P. carinii* pneumonia

	Mild	Moderate	Severe
Symptoms and signs	Increasing exertional dyspnoea, with or without cough and sweats	Dyspnoea on minimal exertion, occasional dyspnoea at rest, fever with or without sweats	Dyspnoea at rest, tachypnoea at rest, persistent fever, cough
Blood gas tensions (room air)	PaO_2 >11·0 kPa	PaO_2 8·0–11·0 kPa	PaO_2 <8·0 kPa
SaO_2 (at rest)	>96%	91–96%	<91%
Chest radiograph	Normal or minor perihilar infiltrates	Diffuse interstitial shadowing	Extensive interstitial shadowing with or without diffuse alveolar shadowing

PaO_2 = partial pressure of oxygen; SaO_2 = arterial oxygen saturation, measured with a transcutaneous pulse oximeter.

Treatment

It is important to assess the severity of the pneumonia in order to choose appropriate treatment.

Intravenous high dose co-trimoxazole remains the "gold standard" treatment. Treatment is for 21 days, given intravenously for the first 10–14 days, diluted in 1 in 25 of 0·9% saline, subsequently orally. Patients with mild disease may be treated with oral co-trimoxazole from the outset. The principal side effects are nausea and vomiting, leucopenia, and rash. Routine use of folic or folinic acid does not prevent leucopenia and may be associated with increased therapeutic failure. Zidovudine should be stopped while co-trimoxazole is being given to avoid profound myelosuppression. Conventionally used doses of co-trimoxazole (20 mg/kg/day of the trimethoprim component) may be excessive: dose reduction to 75% of this dose (to maintain serum trimethoprim concentrations at 5–8 μg/ml) has equivalent efficacy and reduced toxicity.

Treatment of *P. carinii* pneumonia

Choice	Mild	Moderate	Severe
First	Co-trimoxazole	Co-trimoxazole	Co-trimoxazole
Second	Pentamidine i.v. *or* Clindamycin and primaquine *or* Dapsone and trimethoprim	Pentamidine i.v. *or* Clindamycin and primaquine *or* Dapsone and trimethoprim	Pentamidine i.v.
Third	Atovaquone	Atovaquone	Clindamycin and primaquine
Glucocorticoids	Unproven benefit	Of benefit	Of benefit

Pentamidine may be used as an alternative treatment at a dose of 4 mg/kg/day (of the isethionate salt) given diluted in 250 ml 5% dextrose by slow intravenous infusion (over 2 hours); it should not be given by intramuscular injection. The major side effects are hypotension and hypoglycaemia; nephrotoxicity with increases in creatinine and urea concentrations may occur. Dose reduction to 3 mg/kg/day is associated with reduced toxicity but may be less effective. Blood pressure and blood glucose concentrations should be closely monitored. Response to pentamidine (defervescence of fever, reduction in dyspnoea, and improvement in blood gases) may take longer (4–7 days) than intravenous co-trimoxazole.

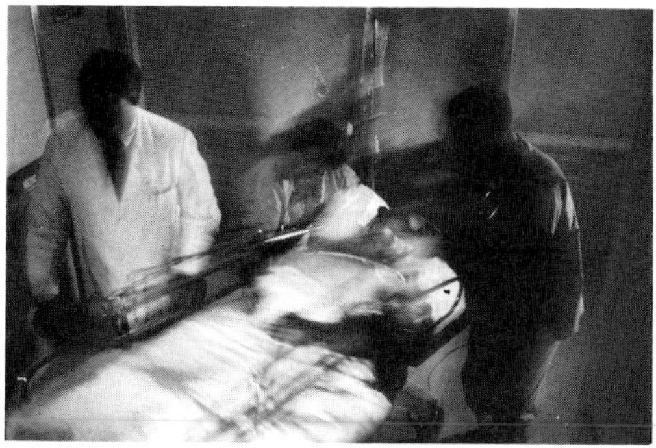

(Zefa-Stockmarket (P Saloutos))

Transfer to the ICU may be necessary if respiratory failure occurs.

Clindamycin–primaquine combination (clindamycin 600 mg × 4/day and primaquine 15 mg/day, both orally) has been used in patients intolerant of, or failing to respond to, co-trimoxazole or pentamidine. Principal side effects are rash, nausea and vomiting, and leuco(neutro) penia.

Dapsone–trimethoprim (100 mg/day dapsone and 20 mg/kg/day trimethoprim) given orally for 21 days is as effective as oral co-trimoxazole in mild to moderate disease and is better tolerated by patients. Side effects include methaemoglobinaemia and hyperkalaemia, nausea, and rash.

Atovaquone given 750 mg × 3/day given orally for 21 days is less effective (and less toxic) than either co-trimoxazole or pentamidine for mild to moderate disease. Absorption from the gut is variable but may be increased if tablets are taken with food.

Nebulised pentamidine is now rarely used to treat pneumocystis pneumonia as there are several other more effective therapies and because this form of treatment does not suppress development of extrapulmonary pneumocystosis.

Adjuvant glucocorticoids for patients with moderate or severe pneumocystis pneumonia reduces the risk of respiratory failure (by up to 50%) and the risk of death (by up to 33%). Glucocorticoids should be started together with specific anti-pneumocystis treatment in any patient presenting with a PaO_2 of ≤9·3 kPa breathing air. In some patients this will be on the basis of a presumptive diagnosis; clearly there will be a need to confirm the diagnosis rapidly. Treatment is with intravenous methylprednisolone 1 g/day for three days, followed by 0·5 g for two days, followed by oral prednisolone initially 40 mg daily tailing off over 10 days. Alternatively prednisolone 40 mg orally twice daily is given for 5 days and then gradually reduced over 21 days.

Prophylaxis of *P. carinii* pneumonia

Primary prophylaxis

- Any HIV positive patient with a CD4 count of $<200\times10^6$/l or persistent unexplained fever or oral candidiasis (irrespective of CD4 count)
- Any HIV positive patient with other AIDS defining illness (Kaposi's sarcoma or toxoplasmosis)

Secondary prophylaxis

- Any HIV positive patient after an episode of *P. carinii* pneumonia

Intensive care

Over 90% of patients respond to treatment and survive their first episode of pneumocystis pneumonia. In those that fail to respond and who develop respiratory failure, mortality is 50%. Transfer to the intensive care unit for mask CPAP ventilation or intubation and mechanical ventilation should be considered in this situation. When considering the appropriateness of intensive care, assess the patient's wishes and those of their partner and relatives as well as the patient's previous and expected quality of life in relation to their HIV disease.

Prophylaxis

HIV-positive patients are at an increased risk of developing pneumocystis pneumonia if their CD4 count is less than 200×10^6/l. Primary prophylaxis (given before an episode) should be given to HIV-positive patients with a CD4 count $<200\times10^6$/l and to HIV-positive patients irrespective of their CD4 count if they are symptomatic with HIV disease (oral candida, fevers, etc.) or if they have other disease definitive for AIDS, such as Kaposi's sarcoma or cerebral toxoplasmosis. Secondary prophylaxis is given to all HIV-positive patients after an initial episode of pneumocystis.

The prophylaxis regimen of choice is co-trimoxazole 960 mg once daily or three times a week. This is well tolerated by patients and does not interact adversely with zidovudine. Co-trimoxazole also protects against bacterial infection and reactivation of cerebral toxoplasmosis. In patients who develop mild to moderate adverse reactions to co-trimoxazole, densitisation may be attempted before changing to alternative therapy. Second line prophylaxis (for those intolerant of, or unwilling to take, co-trimoxazole) is monthly nebulised pentamidine (300 mg given using a Respirgard II or similar nebuliser). There is a higher relapse rate of pneumocystis pneumonia with this regimen compared with that using co-trimoxazole. Some patients who relapse while receiving nebulised pentamidine have atypical chest radiographs with upper zone infiltrates which mimic tuberculosis. Third line prophylaxis is dapsone 100 mg/day (with or without pyrimethamine 25 mg/once weekly).

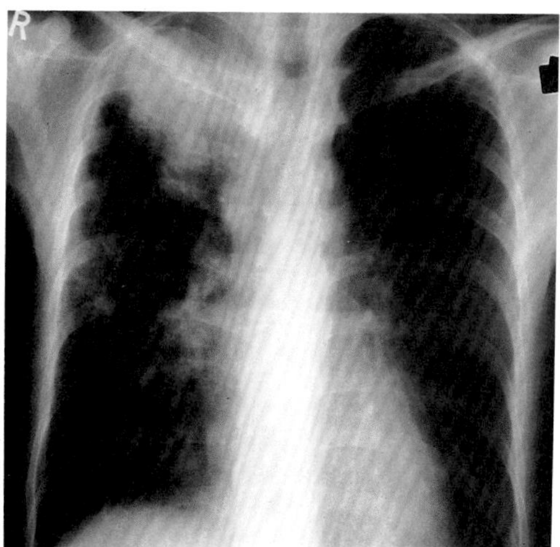

Chest radiograph mimicking tuberculosis in a patient with pneumocystis pneumonia who had received inhaled pentamidine prophylaxis.

Other regimens that are used include i.v. pentamidine 300 mg once every 2–4 weeks and Fansisar (sulfadoxine 500 mg/pyrimethamine 25 mg) 2 tablets once weekly.

Bacterial infections

> The incidence of bronchitis and pneumonia is increased in patients infected with HIV

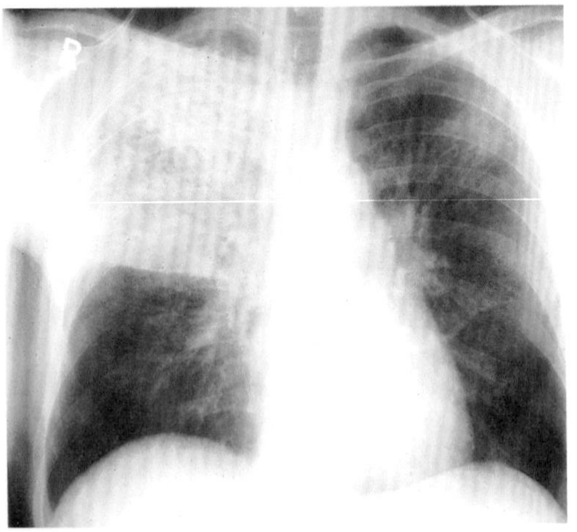

Chest radiograph showing lobar pneumonia due to *Streptococcus pneumoniae*.

Upper respiratory tract infections and pyogenic bacterial infection (sinusitis, bronchitis, and pneumonia) occur more often in HIV-infected individuals than in the general population. Bacterial infections are particularly common in HIV-positive intravenous drug users. The most commonly isolated organisms are *Streptococcus pneumoniae* and *Haemophilus influenzae*. Severe pneumonia due to *Staphylococcus aureus* or Gram negative bacteria such as *Pseudomonas aeruginosa* also occurs, especially in the later stages of AIDS. Respiratory infection may occur with rapid onset, the patient complaining of a cough with or without sputum and fever with chills; patients are frequently bacteraemic. There is a high rate of complications including intrapulmonary abscess formation and empyema. A rapid response usually occurs to treatment with appropriate antibiotics but relapse may occur. Some groups recommend that all HIV positive patients should be immunised with polyvalent pneumococcal polysaccharide vaccine although not all studies have demonstrated effective antibody responses to this agent.

Kaposi's sarcoma

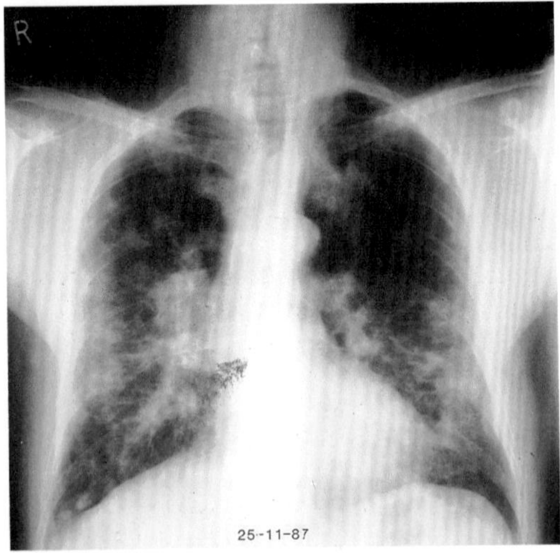

Chest radiograph of pulmonary Kaposi's sarcoma showing multiple pulmonary nodules.

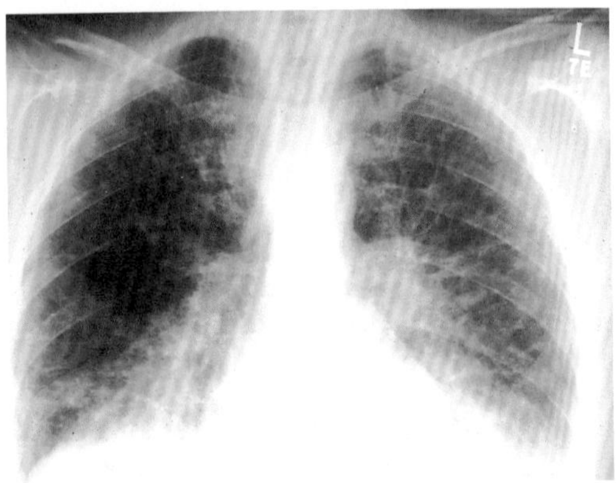

Chest radiogrpah of pulmonary Kaposi's sarcoma showing bilateral pleural effusions and interstitial infiltrates.

Pulmonary Kaposi's sarcoma is the commonest non-infectious pulmonary manifestation of AIDS. Almost all patients with pulmonary Kaposi's sarcoma have mucocutaneous or lymph node Kaposi's sarcoma. Palatal Kaposi's sarcoma (with or without mucocutaneous Kaposi's sarcoma) strongly predicts for the presence of pulmonary Kaposi's sarcoma. Pulmonary Kaposi's sarcoma can affect the pulmonary parenchyma, bronchi, pleura, and hilar/mediastinal lymph nodes. Chest radiographs most frequently show non-specific features, with bilateral interstitial (often nodular) or alveolar infiltrates; more than 40% of patients have pleural effusion and 25% have mediastinal lymph node enlargement. Routine respiratory function tests show decreased lung volumes (FEV_1 and FVC) and decreased carbon monoxide transfer factor; airflow obstruction may occur with extensive Kaposi's sarcoma in the airways.

At fibreoptic bronchoscopy 45% of patients with pulmonary Kaposi's sarcoma have visible endobronchial lesions consisting of multiple, red, or purple, flat or raised lesions. Biopsy is not routinely done as most patients have the diagnosis made by the presence of cutaneous Kaposi's sarcoma, because of the risk of haemorrhage (up to 30% will have a significant bleed) and the low diagnostic yield (<20%) which occurs because of submucous distribution of the tumour.

Transbronchial biopsy also has a low yield of less than 20% due to the patchy nature of parenchymal disease. Histological diagnosis is difficult to make at bronchial or transbronchial biopsy as crush artefact and reactive fibrous tissue have similar appearances. Open lung biopsy has a diagnostic yield of >75%, but this procedure is very invasive and should probably be avoided as patients with pulmonary Kaposi's sarcoma have a poor prognosis.

Treatment

Chemotherapy most often consists of bleomycin 10 IU mg/m^2 and vincristine 2 mg once every three weeks. Liposomal formulations of daunorubicin and doxorubicin may also be used as single-agent chemotherapy. Treatment of pleural effusions (which occcur secondary to Kaposi's sarcoma on the visceral pleura or to mediastinal glands) is problematic. Chemical pleuradesis is rarely successful and radiotherapy has not been shown to be of value.

Tuberculosis

Tuberculosis may speed up the natural history of HIV disease

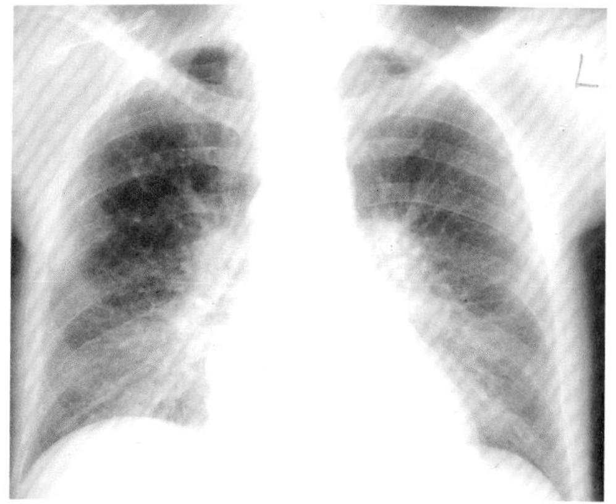

Chest radiograph in a patient with tuberculosis (and CD4 of 100×10^6/l) showing hilar lymphadenopathy.

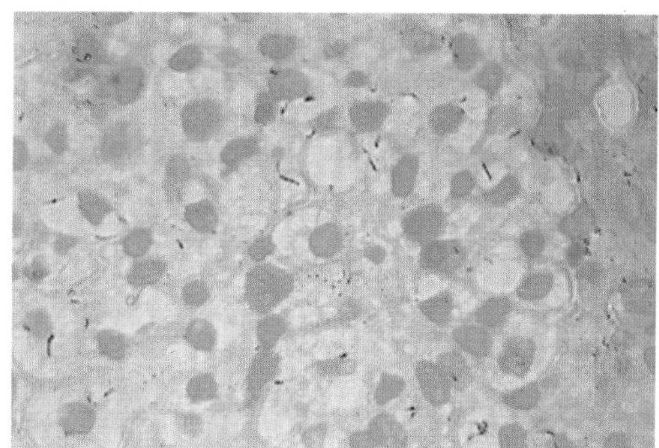

Tissue stained with Ziehl-Neelsen technique showing red staining of mycobacteria ($\times 400$). (Courtesy of Dr Meryl Griffiths.)

Chemoprophylaxis of *M. tuberculosis*

1 HIV positive patient with or without a history of BCG vaccination, negative to tuberculin testing (Heaf 0; Mantoux <5 mm (10 tuberculin units)) and to other recall antigens (Merieux Multitest)

2 CD4 of less than 200×10^6/l

3 History of contact with tuberculosis or history of previous tuberculosis or chest radiographic evidence of previous tuberculosis

Subcommittee of Joint Tuberculosis Committee of the British Thoracic Society *BMJ* 1992;**304**:1231–3.

Unlike opportunistic infections in AIDS tuberculosis is also infectious for healthy individuals. Tuberculosis is a potent stimulator of cell-mediated immunity and so may speed up the natural history of HIV disease. The incidence of tuberculosis is currently increasing in the United States: this is directly attributable to the effects of HIV in certain populations. No increase has occurred yet in Britain, but the unpredictable features of the HIV epidemic in heterosexuals, migrants, and injecting drug users means careful vigilance is required. Tuberculosis can precede development of AIDS, be diagnosed at same time, or occur at any time during established AIDS. Tuberculosis in HIV positive patients is AIDS defining and in Great Britain is a statutorily notifiable disease.

Clinical presentation varies according to the stage of HIV disease. Early on, with relatively well preserved cell mediated immunity, tuberculosis resembles classic adult post-primary disease with upper lobe infiltrates and cavitation; the tuberculin test is usually positive and acid and alcohol fast bacteria (AAFB) are frequently seen when sputum is examined by microscopy. With advanced HIV disease and destroyed cell immunity, presentation is non-specific with fever, weight loss, and fatigue, with or without cough. Patients with low CD4 counts $<150 \times 10^6$/l may also have extrapulmonary disease affecting bone marrow, lymph node, central nervous system, or liver. In the chest the clinical pattern is one of primary infection with hilar and mediastinal adenopathy, diffuse or miliary shadowing; pleural effusions are common. Cavitation occurs rarely and up to 10% of chest radiographs are normal. The tuberculin test is usually negative, sputum (and bronchoalveolar lavage) are often smear negative and culture may also be negative.

Treatment

Clinical response to conventional treatment with isoniazid, rifampicin, and pyrazinamide (with ethambutol if there is primary isoniazid resistance) is good but survival is poor. Treatment with three (or four) drugs should be given for 2 months and then rifampicin and isoniazid for at least 4 further months. Secondary prophylaxis with isoniazid for life is recommended by both American and British Thoracic Societies. HIV-positive patients have a high incidence of adverse drug reactions to antituberculous drugs. Compliance is a problem in some groups, especially injecting drug users, and supervised treatment may be needed. In any HIV-positive patient with AAFB identified from sputum, or an aspirate, or biopsy site, conventional antituberculous treatment should be started. When results of culture are available and if *Mycobacterium avium intracellulare* and not *M. tuberculosis* is identified, treatment should be changed to one of the regimens below.

Multiple drug resistance (MDR) tuberculosis has become a significant clinical problem in the United States in both prison and hospital settings; MDR tuberculosis has been reported in AIDS centres in the UK. Most MDR tuberculosis arises because of inadequate treatment or poor compliance with therapy. Despite treatment, MDR tuberculosis has a poor prognosis in HIV-infected patients and also non-HIV-infected patients and health care workers who acquire MDR tuberculosis.

Primary chemoprophylaxis

An HIV-positive patient with a CD4 count of $<200 \times 10^6$/l regardless of previous BCG vaccination, with a negative tuberculin skin test (Heaf, 0; Mantoux <5 mm (10 tuberculin units)) and negative skin tests to at least two other recall antigens (such as Merieux Multitest) should receive prophylaxis with isoniazid 300 mg daily if they have a history of contact with tuberculosis or have a history, or chest radiographic evidence, of previous tuberculosis. HIV-positive patients with previous BCG vaccination and positive tuberculin reaction (Heaf, 3–4; or Mantoux >10 mm (10 units)) or those with no prior BCG and positive skin tuberculin reaction (Heaf, 1–4; or Mantoux >5 mm (10 units)) should also receive prophylaxis with isoniazid.

Mycobacterium avium intracellulare infection

Symptoms and signs

Fever
Night sweats
Weight loss
Anorexia
Malaise
Anaemia
Hepatomegaly
Chronic diarrhoea
Abdominal pain

Mycobacterium avium intracellulare infection tends to occur at the end of the natural history of HIV disease; it is rare in patients with a count of $>100\times10^6/l$ (CD4 counts are often $<60\times10^6/l$). Up to 50% of HIV-positive patients develop disseminated infection with *M. avium intracellulare* at some stage before death. *M. avium intracellulare* infection reduces survival and causes clinical disease. Symptoms and signs are non-specific and include fever, night sweats, weight loss, anorexia, and malaise; anaemia is common as are hepatomegaly, chronic diarrhoea, and abdominal pain. In the thorax, mediastinal lymphadenopathy is common and, rarely, pneumonic consolidation may occur. The diagnosis of disseminated *M. avium intracellulare* is made from cultures of blood, or biopsy specimen, or aspiration from lymph node, liver, or bone marrow. Bronchoalveolar lavage, sputum, and urine are also frequently positive, but identification of *M. avium intracellulare* from these sites is not diagnostic of disseminated infection.

Treatment of disseminated *M. avium intracellulare*

First line		
Rifabutin	oral	600 mg/day*
or		(450 mg/day if weight <50 kg)
Rifampicin		
+		
Ethambutol	oral	15 mg/kg/day
+		
Clarithromycin	oral	500–1000 mg twice daily
Drug intolerance		
Ciprofloxacin	oral	500 mg twice daily
Clofazimine	oral	100 mg once daily
Refractory symptoms		
Amikacin	i.v.	7·5 mg/kg/day** for 2–4 weeks
Palliative		
Prednisolone	oral	2–3 mg/kg/day

Treatment is for life
* Reduce dose to 300 mg/day if clarithromycin or enzyme inhibitors also used
** Drug concentrations must be monitored

Treatment

No worthwhile response occurs to conventional antimycobacterial treatment. Single-agent treatment is of temporary benefit only; fever, anorexia, and mycobacteraemia rapidly recur. A combination of rifabutin (or rifampicin) with ethambutol and clarithromycin has been shown to improve symptoms and reduce mycobacteraemia. Ciprofloxacin and clofazimine may be used in cases of intolerance. Amikacin may be added for patients with refractory fever and anorexia. Palliative glucocorticoids, such as prednisolone, may be given to patients whose symptoms have not responded to treatment. Treatment is for life; the drug combinations used have high rates of adverse reactions.

Fungal pneumonia

- Cryptococcal pneumonia often part of disseminated infection
- Respiratory symptoms of cough and dyspnoea non-specific
- Chest radiograph may be normal or show diffuse shadowing

Infection with *Cryptococcus neoformans*, *Histoplasma capsulatum*, *Aspergillus fumigatus*, and other fungi is well recognised in HIV-positive patients in the United States and Africa. Infections with these organisms is relatively uncommon in the United Kingdom. Cryptococcal pneumonia often occurs as part of a disseminated infection with fungaemia and meningoencephalitis; respiratory symptoms of cough and dyspnoea are non-specific. The chest radiograph may be normal or show diffuse shadowing which may be nodular. Diagnosis is made by culture of bronchoalveolar lavage or transbronchial biopsy specimen (or blood, bone marrow, or cerebrospinal fluid in disseminated infection). Treatment of cryptococcus infection is with fluconazole 400–600 mg/day or intravenous amphotericin B (up to 0·6 mg/kg/day) and of histoplasma with either amphotericin B or intraconazole 400 mg twice a day. Aspergillus pulmonary infection has a very poor prognosis. It occurs almost exclusively in patients with advanced HIV disease who are either neutropenic or who have received broad spectrum antibiotics.

Lymphoma

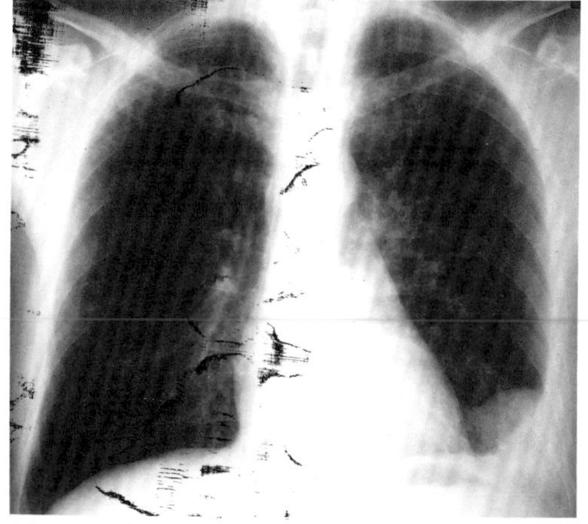

Chest radiograph showing left pleurally based lymphoma.

Lymphoma occurs more often in HIV-positive patients, particularly in those with advanced HIV disease. Most lymphomas are B cell in origin and are of high grade. Intrathoracic disease most frequently occurs in the context of disseminated disease. Symptoms are non-specific. The chest radiograph may show mediastinal lymphadenopathy, pleural lesions, or focal parenchymal abnormalities. The prognosis is poor and there is a high relapse rate after treatment. Mean survival is <1 year, reflecting the advanced stage of HIV disease.

Lymphoid interstitial pneumonitis

Slowly progressive dyspnoea
Cough

In children this condition is common; it is unusual in HIV-infected adults. Parotid enlargement and lymphocytic infiltration of the liver and bone marrow may accompany pulmonary involvement. Patients often present with slowly progressive dyspnoea and cough, symptoms that cannot be distinguished from infection. Examination of the chest may be normal or reveal fine end inspiratory crackles. The chest radiograph usually shows bilateral reticulonodular infiltrates but may show diffuse shadowing and thus mimic *P. carinii* pneumonia. Diagnosis is made by transbronchial biopsy or open lung biopsy. Some patients have been shown to respond to prednisolone 60 mg once a day and others to treatment with zidovudine.

Non-specific pneumonitis

Symptoms are similar to those of *P. carinii* pneumonia

This condition is important as patients present with symptoms and chest radiographic appearances similar to those of *P. carinii* pneumonia. It may also occur when the CD4 count is still normal. Episodes are usually self-limiting but prednisolone may be of benefit. The diagnosis can only be made by biopsy.

Cytomegalovirus

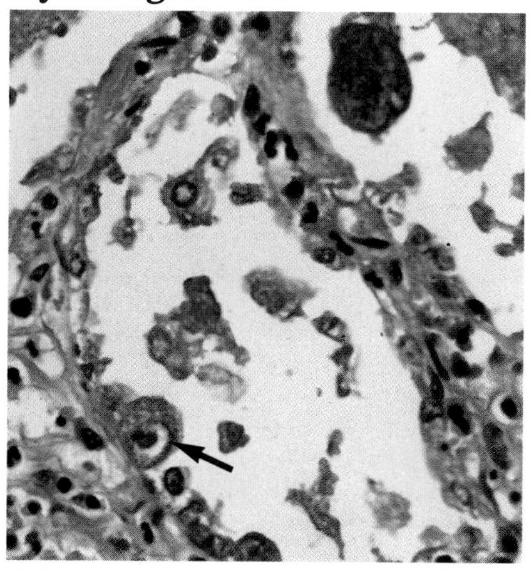

A transbronchial biopsy specimen showing a large eosinophilic nuclear inclusion (arrowed) in a pneumocyte infected with cytomegalovirus (haematoxylin and eosin stain). (Courtesy of Dr Meryl Griffiths.)

Cytomegalovirus (CMV) infection in HIV-positive patients is common and is a well documented cause of retinitis, colitis, adrenalitis, and radiculopathy. In patients with renal allografts and bone marrow transplants, CMV may cause pneumonitis on an immunopathogenic bias and this is frequently fatal.

CMV was originally thought to be an important cause of pneumonitis in patients with AIDS but it is now known that CMV pulmonary infection occurs only rarely in the absence of other pathogens, and its presence does not adversely affect outcome and survival. Treatment with specific anti-CMV treatment such as foscarnet (phosphonoformate) does not seem to improve outcome (as would be expected if CMV was causing the pneumonitis).

7 GASTROINTESTINAL AND HEPATIC MANIFESTATIONS

Ian McGowan, Ian V D Weller

Gastrointestinal symptoms are a common manifestation of HIV infection. Significant clinical problems tend to occur in patients with advanced immunosuppression. The differential diagnosis of gastrointestinal disease is broad and includes opportunistic infection, malignancy, and the effects of medication. Antiviral drugs and antibiotics have gastrointestinal side effects such as nausea, vomiting, and diarrhoea. HIV can be readily detected in mucosal tissue but the direct role of mucosal HIV infection in the cause of clinical disease remains controversial.

This article will focus on the differential diagnosis and management of common gastroenterological syndromes associated with HIV infection. Clinical investigation may not always be appropriate in advanced disease. It is important to counsel patients about the risks and benefits of invasive procedures as many "specific" diagnoses may not be treatable.

Differential diagnosis of HIV-associated gastrointestinal disease

- Infection
- Malignancy
- Medication
- HIV infection

Oral and oesophageal disease

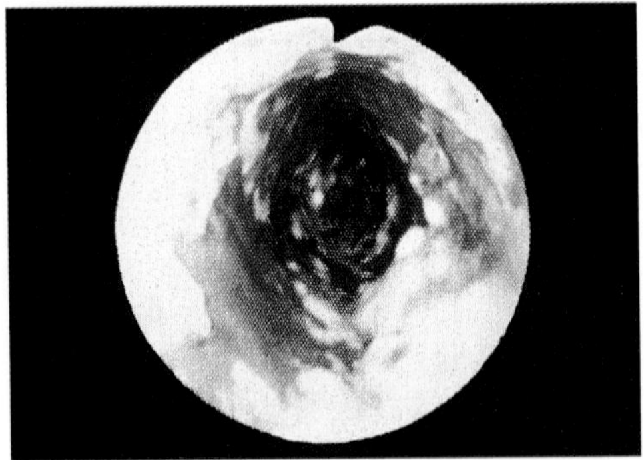

White plaques of oesophageal candidiasis seen at endoscopy.

Oral cavity pain or discomfort are caused by candidiasis, herpetic or aphthous ulceration, periodontal disease, and tumours. Often the diagnosis can be made by simple inspection and appropriate treatment initiated without further investigation. Systemic oral therapy of herpes simplex ulceration and candidiasis is preferred for reasons of efficacy and ease of use. Recurrence is common and, as with many complications of HIV infection, maintenance therapy may be necessary.

About one third of patients develop oesophageal disease. The likelihood of candidiasis is so high that a therapeutic trial with a systemic antifungal agent is indicated before considering further investigation. If symptoms fail to respond, or recur despite adequate maintenance therapy, endoscopy is performed to exclude herpes simplex, cytomegalovirus, or malignant oesophageal ulceration.

Diarrhoea

Infective causes of diarrhoea

- Bacteria
  - campylobacter, salmonella, shigella
  - atypical mycobacteria
  - *Clostridium difficile*
- Protozoa
  - cryptosporidium
  - microsporidia
  - *Isospora belli* and cyclospora
- Viruses
  - cytomegalovirus
  - adenovirus
  - (HIV)

Patients with diarrhoea lasting more than two weeks should be investigated. The diagnostic yield is likely to be highest in patients with CD4 counts $<200\times10^6$/l. Careful microbiological and parasitological examination of multiple stool specimens is the most cost-effective initial investigation. Endoscopy with collection of tissue from the distal duodenum, ascending and descending colon should be performed to exclude cytomegalovirus and occult parasitic infection.

Bacterial infection with *Campylobacter*, *Salmonella* or *Shigella* spp. may present with severe diarrhoeal symptoms and/or bacteraemia. It is important to exclude toxic megacolon with plain abdominal radiography. Organisms are usually sensitive to conventional therapy but drugs may need to be given parenterally. Evidence of atypical mycobacterial infection is found in 60% of patients at necropsy.

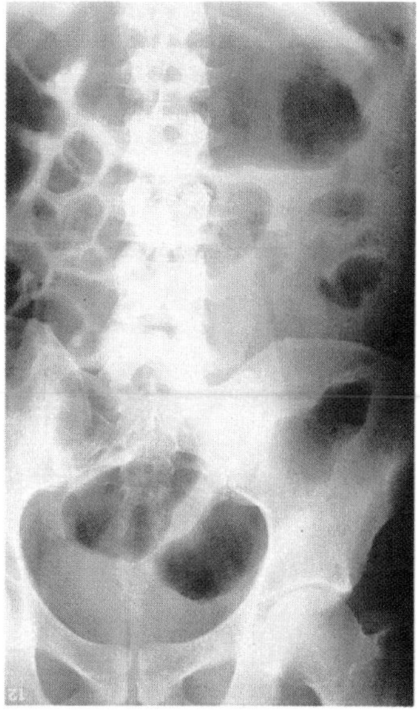

Abdominal radiograph of toxic megacolon secondary to *Shigella flexneri* infection.

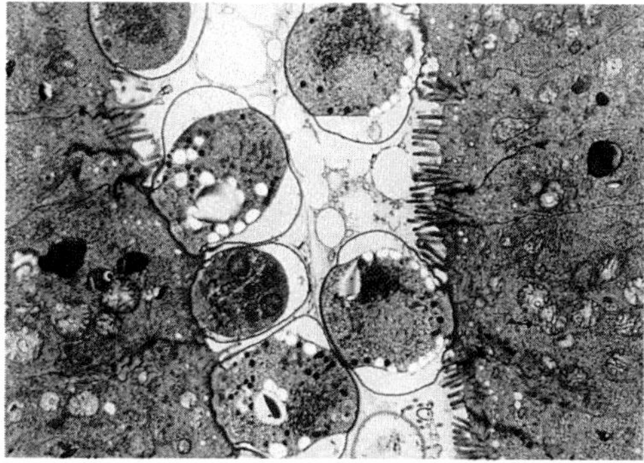

Cryptosporidium on electromicrograph. Developmental stages of cryptosporidium on the surface of enterocytes (note microvilli). The cryptosporidia are surrounded by a parasitophorous vacuole, the outer layers of which are derived from host cell outer membranes.

Treatment of HIV-associated diarrhoea

- Specific
  - antibiotics
  - antivirals
- Fluid replacement
- Antidiarrhoeal agents
  - loperamide
  - diphenoxylate
  - codeine
- Slow release morphine
- Subcutaneous diamorphine

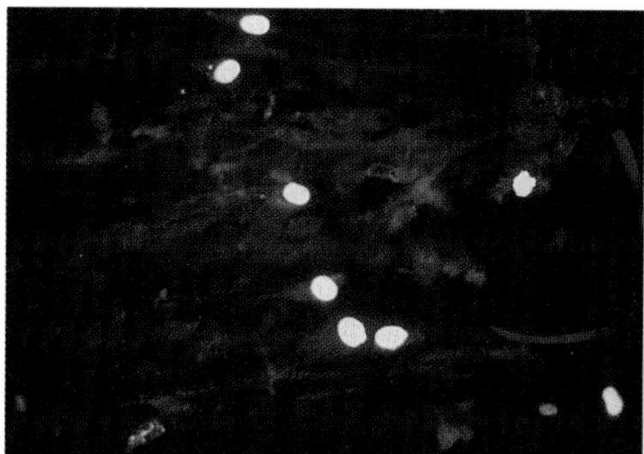

Cytomegalovirus antigen demonstrated by immuno fluorescence microscopy after culturing human fibroblasts with homogenised intestinal tissue.

Gastrointestinal infection may be associated with fever, weight loss, diarrhoea, and malabsorption. Diagnosis can be made by acid fast staining of the stool or biopsy material and by culture. Positive stool culture alone indicates colonisation only. *Mycobacterium tuberculosis* infection of the bowel does occur but is less common. Antibiotic-associated diarrhoea, including pseudomembranous colitis due to *Clostridium difficile*, is occasionally seen in patients with HIV infection and is treated with oral metronidazole or vancomycin.

Cryptosporidium spp. is one of the most common pathogens isolated from HIV-infected patients with diarrhoea. The degree of immunosuppression influences patient prognosis and patients with a CD4 count $>200 \times 10^6$/l may recover spontaneously. Treatment is supportive as no agent has shown convincing efficacy. The organism is heat sensitive and immunosuppressed patients are advised to boil water for drinking purposes.

Microsporidia are also an important cause of diarrhoea as well as being associated with hepatitis, peritonitis, sclerosing cholangitis, sinusitis, and renal failure. Diagnosis is difficult as the spores are only 1·5 μm in diameter. A number of centres have reported successful identification of spores in stool using trichrome and fluorescent stains but morphology is best determined using electron microscopy. Albendazole has shown promise in AIDS patients with microsporidiosis but may only be active against *Encephalitozoon intestinalis* and not *Enterocytozoon bienusi*.

Isospora belli is an infrequent cause of diarrhoea in AIDS patients in the USA and Europe but accounts for up to 25% cases of chronic diarrhoea in patients in tropical and subtropical countries. Response to trimethoprim–sulphamethoxazole has been described.

Cyclospora sp. is the most recent protozoan to be associated with diarrhoea in AIDS. It appears to be more common in the developing world and in returning travellers and like *Isospora belli* appears to be sensitive to trimethoprim–sulphamethoxazole.

Other protozoa including *Entamoeba histolytica* are frequently identified in stools from HIV-infected homosexual men but appear not to be pathogenic.

Cytomegalovirus colitis occurs in less than 5% of patients with AIDS. Symptoms include bloody diarrhoea, abdominal pain, and fever. Sigmoidoscopy may show diffuse erythema and mucosal ulceration. Diagnosis is histopathological and is made on the basis of characteristic intranuclear "owl's-eye" inclusion bodies or detection of CMV antigen with monoclonal antibodies. Treatment is with ganciclovir or foscarnet.

Adenoviruses have been identified by culture and electron microscopy in HIV-infected homosexual men with diarrhoea. No specific treatment is available.

Weight loss and anorexia

Weight loss is a major problem in AIDS and directly influences survival. The causes of weight loss are complex and several factors may coexist in individual patients. Anorexia may occur secondary to drug therapy, opportunistic infection, taste disturbance, or oral discomfort, resulting in inadequate food intake. Malabsorption of fat, lactose, vitamin B12, and bile salts has been demonstrated.

Simple dietary measures such as encouraging smaller, more frequent, meals may be helpful and a wide variety of nutritional supplements are available. Appetite stimulants such as megestrol acetate may be beneficial but weight gain is usually modest. Recombinant human growth hormone, although expensive, may partially reverse HIV-associated weight loss. In patients unable to tolerate oral feeding, enteral and parenteral feeding are alternative forms of nutrition but their efficacy and place in management are still being evaluated. Enteral nutrition offers a safer and cheaper alternative to total parenteral nutrition which is perhaps most useful in patients with severe diarrhoea, nausea, and vomiting, in whom fluid balance and control of symptoms has been difficult.

Hepatitis and cholestasis

Differential diagnosis of liver disease

- Hepatitis or cholestasis
  - *M. avium-intracellulare* complex
  - Drug-induced
  - Viral hepatitis
  - Cytomegalovirus
  - *Mycobacterium tuberculosis*
  - *Cryptococcus*
  - Microsporidia
  - Lymphoma
  - Kaposi's sarcoma
- Biliary disease
  - *Cryptosporidium*
  - Cytomegalovirus
  - Microsporidia
  - Lymphoma
  - Kaposi's sarcoma

Abnormal liver biochemistry and/or hepatomegaly are common clinical problems although frank jaundice is uncommon. The differential diagnosis is wide and may involve the use of serology, abdominal ultrasound, ERCP, and liver biopsy. These latter two diagnostic procedures are clearly invasive and would not be indicated unless treatment of opportunistic infection, malignancy or biliary strictures was contemplated. In the absence of dilatated bile ducts on ultrasound, liver biopsy usually shows a granulomatous hepatitis caused by atypical mycobacteria.

AIDS sclerosing cholangitis presents with right upper quadrant pain, accompanied by a raised alkaline phosphatase. Abdominal ultrasound is abnormal in the majority of patients with biliary tract dilatation. ERCP may demonstrate papillary stenosis, dilatation of the common bile duct and dilatations and strictures with "beading" of the intrahepatic ducts. The disease is commonly associated with cryptosporidiosis, microsporidiosis, or cytomegalovirus infection. Endoscopic sphincterotomy may give pain relief in a proportion of patients with papillary stenosis. Liver function tests do not usually improve, and as it is a late-stage manifestation, the prognosis is poor, with most patients dying from some other HIV-related complication within six months of diagnosis.

HIV infection may alter the natural history of hepatitis B infection in a number of ways. The response rate to hepatitis B vaccination is lower in HIV-infected recipients. Immunodeficiency may favour the establishment of chronic infection following acute infection and HBV replication is increased with a reduction in the rate of spontaneous loss of HBe antigen. In addition, interferon therapy would appear to be less effective in chronic HBV/HIV dual infection.

Hepatitis C virus infection is found primarily in intravenous drug users, although it may also be sexually transmitted. HIV can modify the natural history of HCV infection and patients with HIV/HCV dual infection tend to have more aggressive liver disease.

With the multiple therapies being used in treatment and prophylaxis, a drug-induced hepatitis must always be considered in a patient with AIDS and abnormal liver function tests.

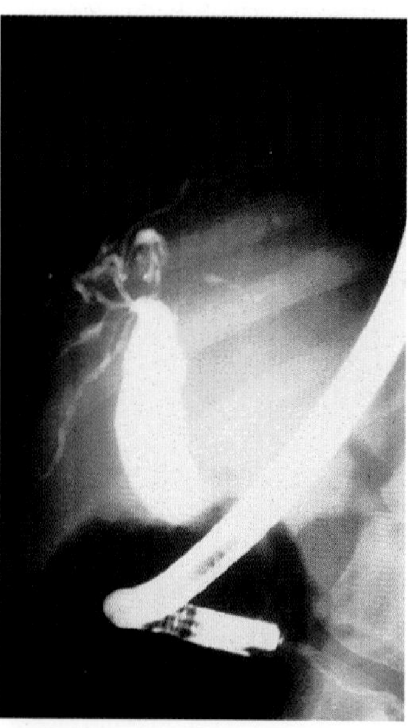

ERCP of AIDS sclerosing cholangitis with intrahepatic biliary tract distortion and dilatation of the common bile duct.

Anorectal disease

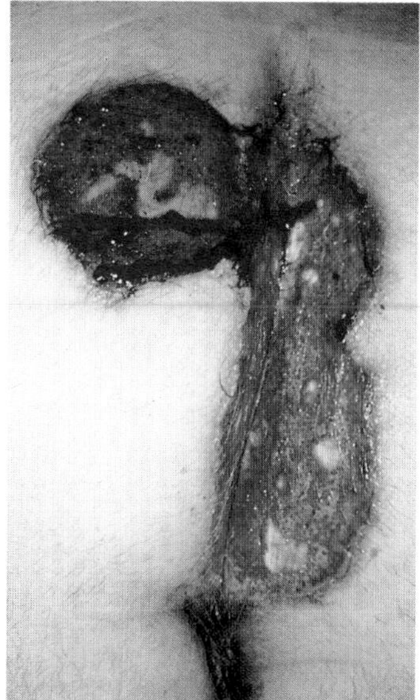

Aciclovir-resistant perianal herpes simplex infection.

Perianal discomfort is often caused by recurrent herpes simplex infection. The diagnosis should be confirmed by viral culture. Patient-initiated intermittent aciclovir can give adequate symptom control in some cases but many patients will require long-term maintenance therapy. Resistance to both aciclovir and ganciclovir has been reported. Foscarnet is then the treatment of choice.

Anal warts are common but rarely cause much in the way of symptoms and should be treated on merit given the absence of any effective antiviral therapy. Anal intraepithelial neoplasia has been described in association with human papillomavirus infection but reports of invasive malignancy are still infrequent.

Patients may present with a mucopurulent proctitis, possible causes of which include recently acquired or long-standing *Neisseria gonorrhoeae* or *Chlamydia trachomatis* infection.

Neoplasia

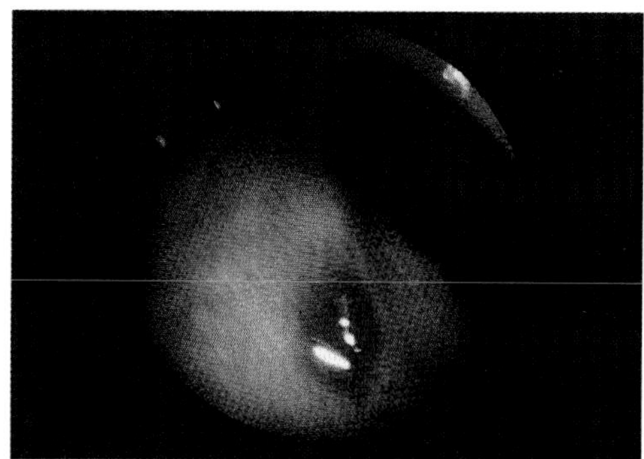

Discrete lesion of Kaposi's sarcoma in the rectum.

Kaposi's sarcoma (KS) is commonly seen in the gastrointestinal tract and occurs in homosexual men more frequently than in patients from other risk groups. A new human herpes virus (HHV8) or Kaposi's sarcoma-associated herpes virus (KSHV) has been recently identified as a likely aetiological agent. KS lesions in the gut have the range seen in the skin, from small telangiectatic lesions, not well shown on contrast studies and only seen at endoscopy, to larger nodular or polypoid lesions. Complications from gastrointestinal disease are unusual, but include ulceration, obstruction, haemorrhage, and diarrhoea.

Lymphoma is much less common than KS. HIV-associated lymphomas are usually high grade non-Hodgkin's type, of B-cell origin. Extranodal involvement is typical and the gut is one of the commonest sites involved.

Acknowledgements

We thank Dr Wilfred Weinstein, UCLA Medical School, Los Angeles for providing the photograph of oesophageal candidiasis and Dr David Casemore, PHLS, Glan Clwyd, North Wales for the electronmicrograph of cryptosporidium.

8 NEUROLOGICAL MANIFESTATIONS

Michael Harrison

About 10% of patients with AIDS present because of neurological problems, but as many as 85% have evidence of disease of the central nervous system at necropsy. The neurological manifestations of AIDS may be caused by opportunistic infections, by tumours, and by the primary neurological effects of HIV. HIV may also, infrequently, cause neurological symptoms in immunocompetent people with HIV infection.

Causes of neurological manifestations

- Opportunistic infections
- Tumours
- Primary effects of HIV

Seroconversion

At the time of seroconversion HIV may cause a self-limiting meningitis, encephalitis, myelitis, or a Guillain–Barré neuritis. There follows a period of good health with no neurological symptoms despite evidence in the cerebrospinal fluid of persistent infection, and over the course of 5–10 years a steady fall in CD4 cell count. In the early asymptomatic years, patients often show a polygammopathy and at this stage an acute or chronic demyelinating polyneuritis or polymyositis can occasionally be seen. Meningitis may also develop with cranial nerve lessons (for example, facial weakness) or long tract signs. The prognosis is usually good.

Neurotropic effects of HIV

At seroconversion, *acute*

- Encephalitis
- Meningitis
- Myelopathy
- Neuropathy

Progression

As CD4 cell counts fall the patients become vulnerable to opportunistic infections, tumours like lymphomas, and conditions that are thought to reflect a direct effect of HIV on the nervous system.

Cryptococcal meningitis

Features of cryptococcal meningitis

- Headache, fever, constitutional upset
- Neck stiffness, photophobia in < third
- Focal signs in 10%
- *Diagnosis*: cryptococcal antigen in cerebrospinal fluid and blood

The commonest cause of meningitis in AIDS is the common soil fungus *Cryptococcus neoformans*. The illness may not resemble a textbook meningitis in that there may be no neck stiffness. Headache, fever and malaise may be the only presenting features, and although the cerebrospinal fluid may contain an elevated protein and cell count and reduced glucose concentration, it may be entirely normal. The diagnosis depends on India ink staining of the cerebrospinal fluid (70% positive), and detection of cryptococcal antigen in the blood and CSF (95–100% positive). Treatment is with amphotericin B and flucytosine, or fluconazole in milder cases. Fluconazole is preferred for lifelong maintenance, to prevent relapse.

Treatment of cryptococcal meningits

Amphotericin B: 0·3–0·5 mg/kg/day i.v. increasing to 1 mg/kg/day
±5-flucytosine: 100 mg/kg/day i.v. increasing to 150 mg/kg/day
or fluconazole: 200–400 mg/day

Cerebral toxoplasmosis

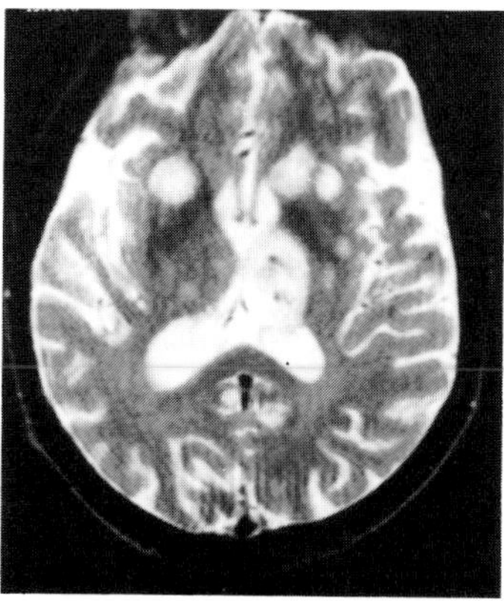

T_2-weighted MRI scan showing multiple rounded or oval abscesses before treatment in cerebral toxoplasmosis.

Features of toxoplasma encephalitis/ abscesses

- Headache, confusion, personality change
- Subacute focal deficit, e.g. hemiplegia
- Seizures
- Fever in less than a third
- *Diagnosis*: CT or MRI and response to treatment

Treatment of toxoplasma encephalitis

Pyrimethamine: 50–100 mg
+sulphadiazine: 4–6 g day
or clindamycin: 600–1200 mg × 4/day
+folinic acid: 15 mg/day

Headache and confusion may also herald the development of focal encephalitis and abscess formation due to toxoplasma infection. This is almost always a reinfection due to loss of immune surveillance in patients who have been exposed to the parasite in their youth. Focal signs develop rapidly and the patients may develop seizures and depressed levels of consciousness. CT and MRI scans show multiple masses which often show ring enhancement and surrounding oedema. The diagnosis is based on the clinical and neuroradiological response to medication with pyrimethamine and sulphonamide or clindamycin. If there is no such response a brain biopsy may be indicated to diagnose the other chief cause of mass lesions, a primary brain lymphoma.

Cerebral lymphoma

Features of lymphomas

- Headache, confusion
- Seizures
- Subacute focal deficit
- *Diagnosis*: CT or MRI, biopsy

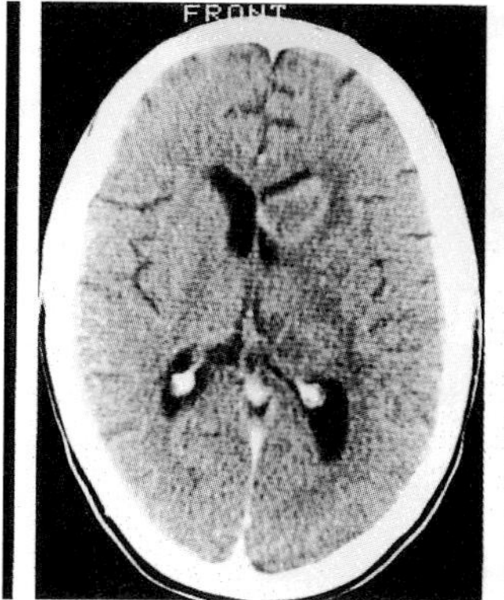

Enhancing right frontal mass lesion due to lymphoma.

These aggressive B cell tumours are rare until immune suppression is severe and CD4 cell counts are extremely low. They are linked to Epstein–Barr virus infection The patients again develop headache, confusion, seizures, and focal deficit. Imaging may be unable to distinguish between lymphoma and toxoplasma abscess, and definitive diagnosis depends on biopsy. Usually lack of response to anti-toxoplasma treatment triggers consideration of biopsy or blind radiotherapy to which these tumours are sensitive. The quality of life can be improved thereby, although the prognosis is very poor because of the patients' vulnerability to infections such as pneumonia.

Progressive multifocal leukoencephalopathy

Features of progressive multifocal leukoencephalopathy

- Progressive focal deficit (hemiplegia, ataxia, aphasia, visual field defect)
- Headache and seizures uncommon
- *Diagnosis*: CT or MRI, JC virus by PCR in CSF or brain biopsy

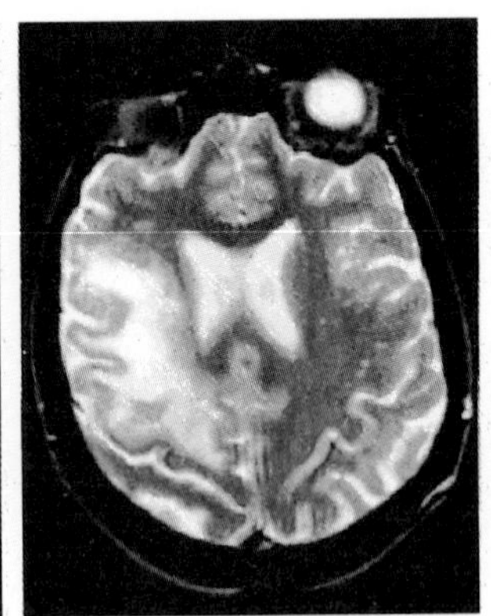

T_2-weighted MRI scan showing large area of high signal in the hemispheric white matter with no mass effect. Biopsy proved progressive multifocal leucoencephalopathy.

Opportunistic viruses include papova viruses like JC virus which is cytopathic for oligodendroglia and causes demyelination of white matter tracts. This condition, called progressive multifocal leukoencephalopathy, presents as a focal deficit with little headache and no early change in conscious level, as there is no mass effect. CT and MRI scans show areas of abnormal signal in the white matter with little or no mass effect, and little or no enhancement. There is as yet no proven treatment. Survival is quite varied from a few months to about two years. The diagnosis is made on the clinical picture and imaging, and can often be confirmed by the identification of JC virus DNA in the CSF. Attempts to improve patients' immune state by aggressive antiretroviral treatment are the current best therapeutic measures.

Other viruses

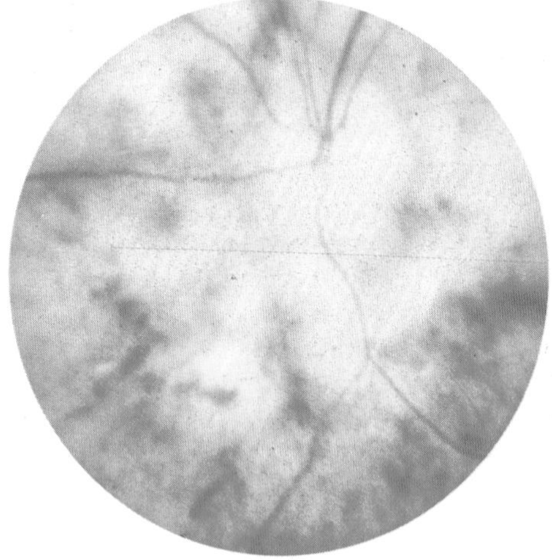

Haemorrhagic retinitis due to cytomegalovirus.

Cytomegalovirus (CMV) can be responsible for encephalitis, a brain stem syndrome, or a lumbosacral radiculopathy causing pain and weakness in the legs with loss of sphincter control. Diagnosis in all of these cases is difficult but viraemia and associated CMV retinopathy can be sufficiently suggestive to warrant a trial of therapy with ganciclovir or foscarnet for the neurological condition as well as for the retinal infection. CMV may play a role in the painful neuropathy described below but its treatment has yet to be proved to benefit that condition. Herpes simplex and zoster cause occasional cases of meningoencephalitis and myelitis.

HIV-1-associated cognitive motor complex

Features of HIV-1-associated cognitive motor complex

- Personality change, apathy, flat effect
- Loss of memory and concentration
- Unsteadiness, hyperreflexia, extensor plantar responses
- *Diagnosis*: neuropsychology and exclusion of other causes or biopsy. CT/MRI show atrophy and white matter change

As many as 80% of patients dying of AIDS have histological evidence of an encephalopathy varying from a bland loss of cortical neurones through a pallor of the white matter with varying degrees of gliosis to a frank giant cell encephalitis. The clinical counterpart of these changes may be undetectable or, in up to a third of AIDS patients, a dementing illness, with or without motor and behavioural changes, originally referred to as the AIDS dementia complex. This is usually a late feature although occasionally it is the first sign of severe immunosuppression and is the AIDS-defining illness. Patients lose interest, become apathetic and emotionally flat with poor concentration and memory. The differential diagnosis includes the psychological effects of bereavement, anxiety and depression and the toxic and metabolic effects of pneumonia, hypoxia, and medication. Neuropsychological testing is

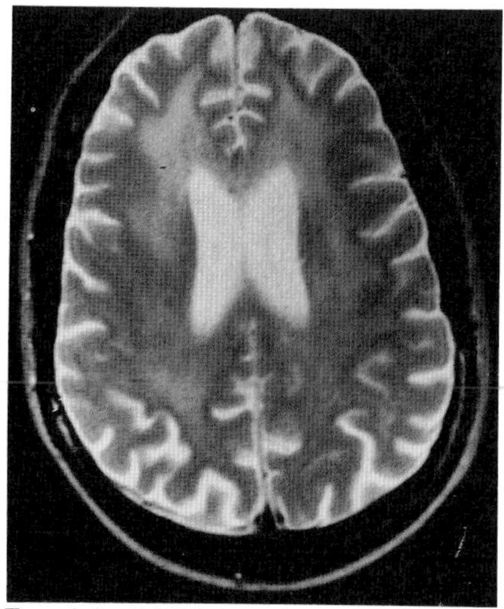

T_2-weighted MRI scan showing "milky" hyperintensity of the hemispheric white matter in a demented patient.

frequently necessary to complete the assessment. Motor signs with hyperreflexia, mild ataxia, and extensor plantars support an organic explanation, as do imaging signs of cerebral atrophy and MR changes in the white matter. The dementia may progress rapidly, the patient becoming mute with terminal decorticate posturing, or may appear to plateau with only a modest degree of cognitive impairment.

Myelopathy, peripheral neuropathy, and myopathy

Vacuolar myelopathy

- Symptoms
  - paraesthesiae
  - leg weakness
  - loss of sphincter control
- Signs
  - paraparesis
  - ± spasticity
  - ± ataxia
  - sensory level unusual

Peripheral neuropathy

- Distal
- Symmetrical
- Dysaesthesiae
- ± Weakness
- ± Distal atrophy

Types of peripheral neuropathy

- Early
  - acute demyelinating = Guillain–Barré
- Early/late
  - chronic demyelinating
- Late
  - mononeuritis multiplex
  - painful sensory axonal iatrogenic (for example, ddI, ddC)

Types of myopathy

- Early
  - polymyositis
- Late
  - HIV myopathy
  - zidovudine myopathy
  - *Diagnosis*: electromyogram, creatine kinase, biopsy, therapeutic trial

Vacuolar myelopathy

Necropsies also suggest that the spinal cord is affected in perhaps 25% of patients with AIDS. The clinical signs of a spastic paraparesis with ataxia and loss of sphincter control are, however, much rarer.

Peripheral neuropathy

Up to 30% of patients with stage IV disease develop an axonal peripheral neuropathy which mostly affects sensory fibres with pain in the feet and legs. The ankle jerks are lost and a stocking distribution of sensory loss is found; the diagnosis is confirmed by nerve conduction studies. Pain relief is the main therapeutic problem as associated motor disability is unusual. Autonomic involvement is usually asymptomatic. The new antiretrovirals ddI and ddC can cause a painful neuropathy and this can be a reason for stopping treatment. A few patients develop a mononeuritis multiplex due to vasculitis which can be self-limiting or need a trial of steroids.

Myopathy

Complaints of weakness about the hips and shoulders suggest muscle involvement. There is a clinical spectrum from muscle pain through mild weakness to a disabling myopathy with biopsy evidence of fibre necrosis. In some patients there appears to be a mitochondrial defect due to prolonged treatment with zidovudine and symptoms, and elevated creatine kinase levels respond to a change to alternative antiretroviral drugs. A very similar syndrome was recorded before the introduction of zidovudine, however, and this may respond to steroids. If signs of a myopathy do not reverse on stopping zidovudine, steroids should be tried for a period of several months.

9 TREATMENT OF INFECTIONS AND ANTIVIRAL AGENTS

Ian V D Weller, I G Williams

The treatment of HIV infection can be largely divided into:

- measures that either treat or prevent (prophylaxis) its complications, namely opportunistic infections, and tumours
- specific antiviral agents that inhibit viral replication.

Treatment

- of complicating infections
- of the virus itself

Most of the opportunistic infections are due to reactivation of latent organisms in the host or in some cases to ubiquitous organisms to which we are continuously exposed. In general the treatment of these infections suppresses rather than eradicates the organisms, so relapse is common when treatment is stopped. The side effects of many of the drugs used complicate the long-term treatment that is needed.

Antiviral treatment for HIV became possible in the spring of 1987 when zidovudine (AZT), the first 2′3′-dideoxynucleoside analogue reverse transcriptase (RT) inhibitor, became available for use in patients with symptomatic disease. Since then there have been advances in treatment with the development of new nucleoside and non-nucleoside RT inhibitors, proteinase inhibitors and the proven clinical efficacy of combination therapy.

This chapter will cover some of the treatments and infections previously described in the other parts of the book in an attempt to bring all of these together in a comprehensive manner.

Protozoal infections

Pneumocystis carinii pneumonia (PCP)

There have been considerable advances in the diagnosis, treatment and prophylaxis of PCP. Although it has been recently recognised as being more like a fungus, it is considered under protozoa here. Clinical suspicion is aroused early in patients who are under regular medical supervision, leading to earlier diagnosis. Techniques of diagnosis are now less invasive (sputum induction with nebulised saline), which may obviate the need for bronchoscopy, but its diagnostic sensitivity is lower. The use of lavage alone at bronchoscopy avoids transbronchial biopsy with its complications of haemorrhage and pneumothorax. Exercise oximetry and alternative imaging techniques with radiolabelled compounds are also being used in diagnosis. Monoclonal antibodies to pneumocystis proteins may improve diagnostic sensitiviy compared with conventional staining techniques. Sensitive DNA probes for pneumocystitis have been developed but these have yet to reach the bedside.

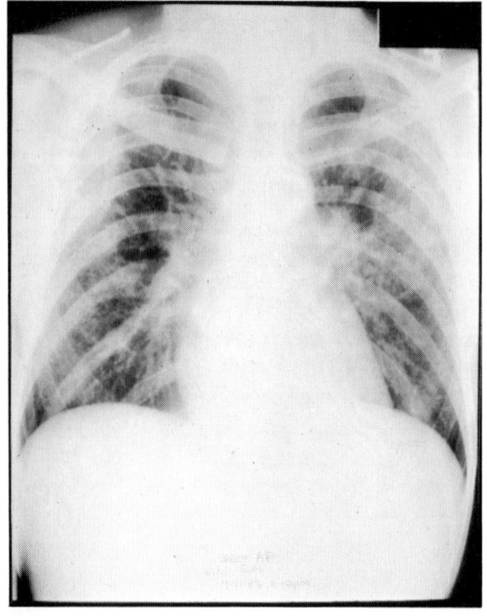

Chest X-ray appearances of *Pneumocystis carinii* pneumonia showing interstitial infiltrates.

High-dose intravenous co-trimoxazole for 2–3 weeks remains a standard first choice regimen for severe PCP, but once fevers and symptoms have settled and blood gas values have improved the drug can be given by mouth. Side effects are common, typically after 7–10 days. If they prevent co-trimoxazole treatment from being continued the drug should be replaced by either intravenous pentamidine or a combination of clindamycin and primaquine. Pentamidine is as effective as co-trimoxazole but has side effects that can be life threatening and should be given by slow intravenous infusion with careful monitoring. In patients with moderate or mild PCP, a combination of clindamycin and primaquine has proven clinical efficacy and is an alternative first choice for those patients who have a previous history of severe co-trimoxazole hypersensitivity. Side effects of rash and diarrhoea are frequent.

A review of clinical trials of the use of high-dose clinical corticosteroids in patients with severe hypoxaemia has led to a consensus that they are beneficial in terms of reducing both morbidity and mortality.

Alternative second-line therapies include trimetrexate with folinic acid or Atovaquone, a hydroxy-naphthoquinone but its efficacy has only been established in mild to moderate *P. carinii* infection. Like trimetrexate it is probably less effective than co-trimoxazole but it is less toxic. Its bioavailability is reduced because of its low aqueous solubility and slow and irregular absorption. Preparations with better bioavailability are being assessed. Other choices include dapsone with trimethoprim and difluoromethylornithine (Eflornithine), which has been used in patients who fail to respond to conventional treatment (salvage therapy).

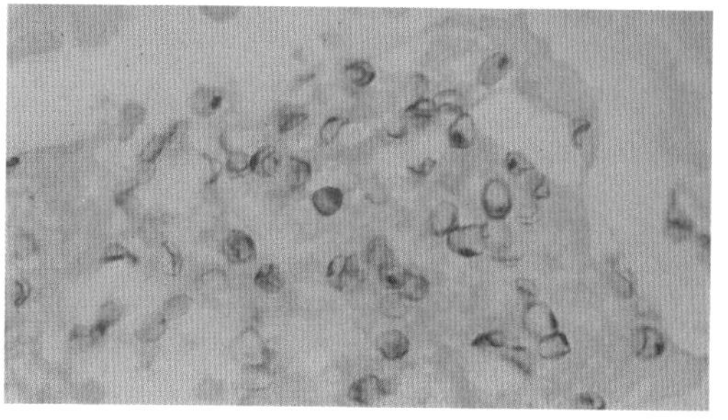

Cysts of *P. carinii* pneumonia in bronchial lavage specimen.

Prophylaxis for PCP is essential after a first attack (secondary prophylaxis) but is also recommended for all patients once their CD4 cell counts fall below 200×10^6/l (primary propylaxis). The risk of a first episode PCP below this CD4 count level is estimated to be 18% at 12 months for those who are asymptomatic rising to 44% for those who have early symptomatic disease (for example, oral candida, fever). Co-trimoxazole 960 mg given by mouth daily or three times per week is the most effective agent. In patients who are intolerant, alternative regimens include oral dapsone 100 mg with pyrimethamine 25 mg daily or three times per week, or nebulised pentamidine. The dosage of the latter depends on the nebuliser system used: with a Respirgard II nebuliser the recommended regimen is 300 mg every 4 weeks. In patients with more advanced disease and CD4 counts $< 100 \times 10^6$/l, 300 mg given every two weeks should be considered in view of the high failure rate of the monthly regimen.

Although clinical trials have shown greater efficacy for co-trimoxazole compared to other regimens there is a high rate of discontinuation owing to side effects. Desensitisation regimens are used with the aim of reducing the rate of intolerance but there is uncertainty about their efficacy and which regimen is best.

P. carinii pneumonia treatment

Drug	*Duration*	*Side effects*	*Comments*
Co-trimoxazole (trimethoprim component 20 mg/kg/day) intravenously or orally daily in divided doses	14–21 days	Nausea, vomiting, fever, rash, marrow suppression	
or pentamidine isethionate 4 mg/kg/day as a slow intravenous infusion	14–21 days	Hypotension, hyper- and hypoglycaemia renal failure, hepatitis, marrow suppression, nausea, vomiting, cardiac arrhythmias	80% of patients will respond to treatment
High dose steroids, such as prednisolone 40–60 mg orally daily	5 days then tapering over 14–21 days		In severe disease optimal dose not determined
Trimethoprim 20 mg/kg intravenously or orally daily in divided doses and dapsone 100 mg orally daily	14–21 days	Rash, nausea, methaemoglobinaemia marrow suppression	Possible bi-directional pharmacokinetic interaction raising plasma concentrations
Clindamycin 600–900 mg 6–8 hourly orally or intravenously and primaquine 15–30 mg orally daily	14–21	Rash, nausea, vomiting, marrow suppression, methaemoglobinaemia, haemolysis	
Trimetrexate 45 mg/m^2 intravenously and folinic acid 30–80 mg/m^2 daily	14–21 days	Raised transaminases, rashes, marrow suppression	
Atovaquone 750 mg three times a day	14–21 days	Rash, raised transaminases	Poor bioavailability
Difluoromethylornithine (Eflornithine) 400 mg/kg daily	14–21 days	Bone marrow suppression	

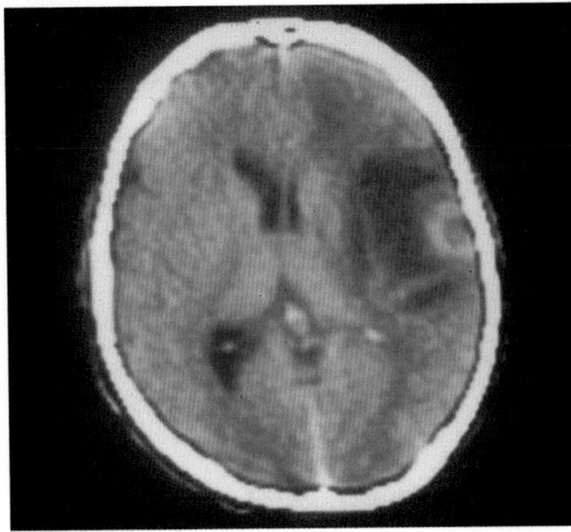

CT scan showing ring-enhancing lesion of cerebral toxoplasmosis surrounded by cerebral oedema (dark area).

Toxoplasmosis

Cerebral toxoplasmosis is the commonest manifestation of toxoplasma infection. As toxoplasmosis is the most common cause of ring-enhancing lesions on contrast CT brain scans a presumptive diagnosis is usually made and treatment started. The condition responds well if treatment is started early, and a combination of sulphadiazine 4–6 g/day and pyrimethamine 50–100 mg/day (both by mouth in divided doses with folinic acid 15 mg/day) is the treatment of choice. Side effects may prevent continued use of sulphadiazine, and clindamycin 600–1200 mg four times a day has been shown to be an effective alternative in controlled studies.

Corticosteroids are sometimes used in addition to first-line treatment to reduce symptomatic cerebral oedema, but a clinical and radiological response seen after two weeks of treatment may be due solely to the corticosteroid effect rather than the antitoxoplasma treatment. A presumptive diagnosis of toxoplasma may therefore be made, although the underlying lesion may be due to something else, such as lymphoma or another infection. Relapse is common after treatment is stopped, and maintenance treatment should continue indefinitely.

Atovaquone 750 mg four times a day and the new macrolides, clarithromycin 2 g/day and azithromycin, both given with pyrimethamine 75 mg/day, have also been effective in small uncontrolled studies.

The most appropriate regimen for secondary prophylaxis has not been determined but treatment doses of either sulphadiazine and pyrimethamine or clindamycin and pyrimethamine are usually halved.

Of patients with positive toxoplasma serology and a CD4 count of $<100 \times 10^6$/l, approximately one in three will develop cerebral toxoplasmosis within 12 months without prophylaxis. Primary prophylaxis in patients with positive serology with a CD4 count of $<200 \times 10^6$/l is therefore recommended. Co-trimoxazole or dapsone with pyrimethamine have been shown to reduce the incidence of toxoplasmosis compared to patients taking nebulised pentamidine for prophylaxis against PCP. Similarly atovaquone might be expected to provide prophylaxis for both if adequate concentrations in the cerebrospinal fluid are obtained with a new formulation; and the new macrolides, clarithromycin and azithromycin, might be anticipated to provide broad spectrum prophylaxis for toxoplasmosis, atypical mycobacterial, and bacterial infections, but bacterial resistance might limit their use in this situation.

Treatment of toxoplasmosis

- *First line*

  Sulphadiazine 4–6 g/day or clindamycin 600–1200 mg 4 × per day
  +
  Pyrimethamine 50–100 mg/day
  +
  Folinic acid 15 mg/day

- *Alternatives*

  Clarithromycin 2 g/day *or*
  Azithromycin and pyrimethamine 50–100 mg/day *or*
  Atavoquone 750 mg 4 × per day

Cryptosporidiosis and other protozoa

The reported successes in *cryptosporidiosis* with a variety of treatments are still anecdotal. Symptoms and excretion of cysts may be intermittent. Responses have been described after treatment with a variety of agents including spiramycin, erythromycin, diclazuril, letrazuril, hyperimmune bovine colostrum, paromomycin, azithromycin, and subcutaneous somatostatin. Atovaquone is also being assessed.

Symptomatic treatment with codeine phosphate, loperamide, and other drugs, together with fluid, electrolyte and nutritional support may be the only effective measure.

With no effective treatment it is important that patients avoid possible exposure in water supplies particularly at times of documented outbreaks. Although unproven, measures that may be considered for patients with CD4 counts $<200 \times 10^6$/l include point of use filters, or boiling water for more than one minute.

In *microsporidiosis* there have been anecdotal reports of symptomatic improvement with albendazole 400 mg twice a day or metronidazole 500 mg three times a day. *Isosporiasis* is less common and appears to respond to cotrimoxazole 960 mg four times a day, but relapses occur in 50% of cases.

Diarrhoea often occurs in the absence of recognised pathogens in the stool, and metronidazole has relieved symptoms in some cases.

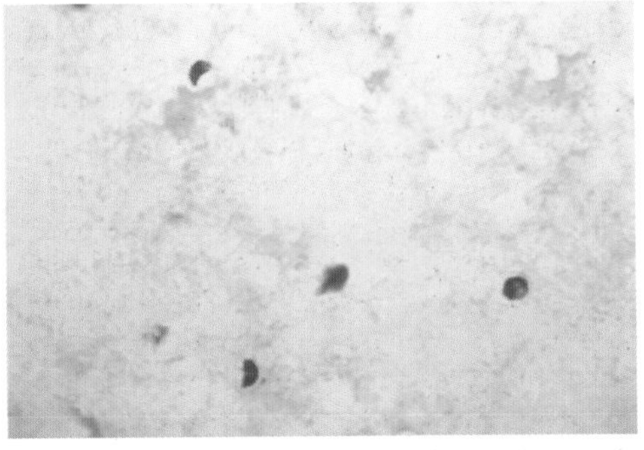

Cryptosporidium.

Viral infections

Viral opportunistic infections

Infection	Drug	Duration	Side effects	Comments
Herpes simplex				
Treatment	Aciclovir 200 mg 5 times a day orally or 5–10 mg/kg 8 hourly intravenously	5–7 days		Duration may be extended in severe infections
Prophylaxis	Aciclovir 200 mg 4 times a day	Indefinite		May be possible to reduce frequency
Cytomegalovirus				
Treatment	Ganciclovir 5 mg/kg twice a day intravenously	14–21 days	Neutropenia, anaemia	Marrow suppression potentiated with zidovudine
	Foscarnet (phosphonoformate) 180 mg/kg daily intravenously	14–21 days	Renal impairment, hypomagnesaemia, hyper- and hypocalcaemia, hyper- and hypophosphataemia, hypokalaemia, gastrointestinal, genital ulcers	Dose must be adjusted according to renal function
Maintenance	Ganciclovir 5 mg/kg once daily intravenously or 1 g × 3/day orally	Indefinite	As above	Maintenance indwelling central line required with intravenous ganciclovir and foscarnet
	Foscarnet 90 mg/kg daily intravenously	Indefinite	As above	Combination of both drugs may be used as maintenance

Acyclic analogues of 2′ deoxyguanosine

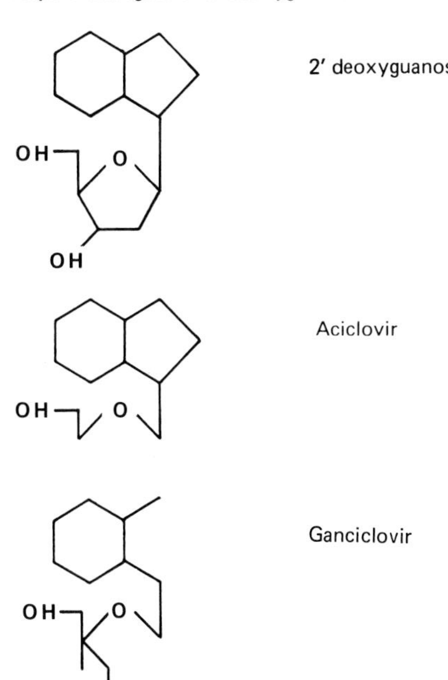

Severe mucocutaneous and systemic infections with herpes simplex virus are best treated with aciclovir. Prophylaxis is used after severe infection and in patients with increasing severity and frequency of recurrences. These recurrences can be a prelude to the chronic persistent mucocutaneous ulceration characteristic of AIDS.

Varicella zoster virus infections are usually treated with high dose aciclovir given by mouth. However, dissemination of infection from dermatomal zoster is unusual even without treatment.

Valaciclovir is a pro-drug of aciclovir which has been used in the treatment of herpes zoster and herpes simplex infections of skin and mucous membranes. Valaciclovir is an L-valine ester of aciclovir that is rapidly converted to aciclovir after oral administrtion. The antiviral spectrum and mode of action is therefore the same as aciclovir. Acyclovir has, however, a low oral bioavailability (about 15–20%). Valaciclovir has three or four times the oral bioavailability of aciclovir.

Famciclovir is a diacetyl ester of 6-deoxy penciclovir which has been used in the treatment of herpes zoster and genital herpes infections. Famciclovir is metabolised to penciclovir in the intestinal wall and liver. Penciclovir and aciclovir have a similar antiviral spectrum.

Aciclovir-resistant herpes simplex and varicella zoster viral infections are emerging as clinically important problems. Both resistant infections have been successfully treated with foscarnet. Topical trifluorothymidine has also been used.

Reactivation of cytomegalovirus infection tends to occur when CD4 cell counts are persistently $<50 \times 10^6$/l. Ganciclovir (an acyclic analogue of deoxyguanosine) and foscarnet (phosphonoformate, a pyrophosphate analogue, which inhibits polymerase enzymes), are both used for the treatment of cytomegalovirus retinopathy and gastrointestinal disease. Both drugs arrest progression of retinitis in most patients but maintenance treatment is required to delay the time to further relapse. The role of maintenance treatment in gastrointestinal disease is less clear. The major side effect of ganciclovir is neutropenia. Foscarnet is not as well tolerated as ganciclovir and it produces reversible renal failure and electrolyte disturbances. Careful and frequent monitoring is required which complicates outpatient management. A study comparing ganciclovir with foscarnet for initial treatment and long-term maintenance in cytomegalovirus (CMV) retinitis found no difference between the drugs in their ability to delay progression of disease but there was a survival advantage in those patients treated with foscarnet: the reasons for this are unclear. Combination therapy with the two drugs may be superior to either alone in preventing further progression of CMV disease in those who have relapsed on maintenance therapy. Ganciclovir is active against herpes simplex virus so patients with frequent recurrences do not require concurrent aciclovir treatment.

Granulocyte colony-stimulating factor (GCSF) can be used to counteract the severe neutropenia associated with ganciclovir induction treatment. Intravitreal implants of ganciclovir or intraocular injections of ganciclovir or foscarnet have also been used, but there may be an increased risk of retinal detachment and this localised delivery of the drug would not be expected to have activity against CMV infection elsewhere including disease in the other eye. More recently studies of the drug cidofovir (a nucleoside analogue with potent *in vitro* activity against herpes viruses) have shown a delay in progression of disease and time to relapse in patients who have previously failed ganciclovir and foscarnet. Cidovofir is given once weekly (5 mg/kg) for two weeks as induction therapy and then every two weeks at the same dose thereafter as maintenance therapy. Further clinical trials are under way. The main side effect is nephrotoxicity.

Ganciclovir is poorly absorbed but an oral preparation at a daily dose of 3 g is available and initial trials in maintenance therapy have not detected a large difference when compared to the drug given intravenously. Furthermore, the inconvenience and rates of infection associated with indwelling intravenous lines makes oral maintenance therapy an attractive option. The oral preparation has also been investigated as primary prophylaxis against CMV retinitis but the results of two large clinical trials are conflicting and in view of the high cost, this has not gained much acceptance in routine clinical practice.

Fungal infections

Fungal opportunistic infections

Infection	*Drug*	*Duration*	*Side effects*	*Comments*
Candidiasis				
Local treatment	Nystatin oral suspension pastilles, miconazole oral gel, or amphotericin lozenges all 4–6 times a day	As required		Relapse common, many patients require systemic treatment
Systemic treatment	Ketoconazole 200 mg/day orally	1–2 weeks	Nausea (less if taken with food), abnormal liver function tests, hepatitis, thombocytopenia, rash	Relapse common on cessation of treatment. Maintenance therapy may be required
	Fluconazole 50–200 mg/day	1–2 weeks	Nausea, abnormal liver function tests	As above
	Itraconazole capsules or solution 200 mg/day	1–2 weeks	Nausea, abnormal liver function tests	
Cryptococcosis				
Treatment	Amphotericin B at least 0·3 mg/kg/day ± flucytosine 150 mg/kg/day in four doses	6 weeks	Nausea, vomiting, rash, bone marrow suppression, renal impairment, hypocalcaemia	Relapse may occur, maintenance needed
	or			
	fluconazole 800 mg on days 1–3, 400–800 mg/day daily thereafter		As above	As above

Dermatophytic fungal infections respond well to imidazole creams. Oral candida is often asymptomatic in its early stages and may not require treatment. In more severe infections local treatment with frequent nystatin suspension, or pastilles, or amphotericin lozenges can be used. Systemic treatment with oral ketoconazole or fluconazole daily is required for more severe oropharyngeal and oesophageal candidiasis. Long-term maintenance treatment may be required to prevent recurrences, and liver function tests should be monitored. Clinical resistance to treatment can occur and in the case of fluconazole may be related to emerging *Candida* species that are less sensitive to fluconazole, or to *Candida albicans*—resistant strains. Intermittent rather than maintenance therapy may be a more appropriate strategy to reduce this risk but has yet to be assessed in a large controlled trial. Itraconazole solution has been found useful in cases of clinical resistance and this may be related to its topical action, better absorption, and greater spectrum of activity.

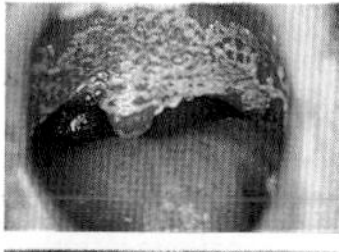

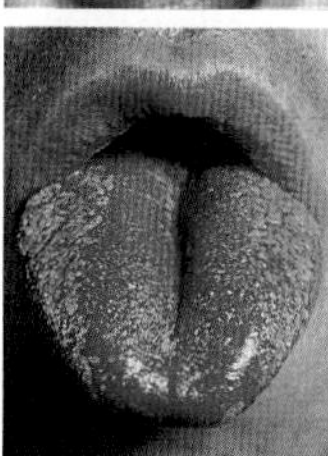

Oral candidiasis.

Vulvovaginal candidiasis can be a recurrent problem in women and should be treated either with topical agents (clotrimazole or miconazole pessaries and cream) or, if chronic and refractory, by oral ketoconazole or fluconazole.

Cryptococcal meningits is treated with either fluconazole or amphotericin B with or without flucytosine. A large comparative study has shown that the overall mortality was similar in both treatment groups. However, there were more early deaths in the fluconazole group, and amphotericin sterilised the cerebrospinal fluid more rapidly, but fluconazole was better tolerated. There was a 20% mortality and the factors predictive of death were an abnormal mental state, a cryptococcal antigen titre >1024 and a white cell count $<0{\cdot}02\times10^9/l$ in the cerebrospinal fluid. Physicians will probably therefore prefer to treat patients with these poor prognostic markers with amphotericin rather than fluconazole. With a 20% mortality irrespective of what treatment is used, it is clear that improvements in treatment are required.

Cryptococcal meningitis treatment

- Fluconazole
  or
  Amphotericin B $\pm$ flucytosine
- Maintenance treatment required

Maintenance treatment is required, without it relapse is common. Fluconazole (200 mg/day) was more effective than amphotericin B (1 mg/kg/week) in a large randomised study. The comparative efficacy of higher doses of amphotericin maintenance treatment is unknown. Liposomal preparations of amphotericin B may be useful particularly in patients at risk of renal toxicity. Controlled studies of high doses of fluconazole suggest greater efficacy but this needs to be confirmed.

Amphotericin B is still the mainstay of treatment of other systemic fungal infections. Itraconazole has shown to be effective in induction and maintenance treatment of disseminated histoplasmosis.

Bacterial infections

Tuberculosis in HIV infection is treated in the standard way with isoniazid and rifampicin plus either pyrazinamide or ethambutol. Rifampicin is a potent enzyme inducer and increases the metabolism of drugs such as oral contraceptives, dapsone, fluconazole, ketoconazole, and anticonvulsants. Furthermore, ketoconazole inhibits the absorption of rifampicin—if both drugs are given together blood concentration of both drugs are reduced. Although extrapulmonary disease is more common in HIV seropositive patients than in uninfected controls, the responses to treatment appear similar in the developed world if patients are compliant. Over the last few years there have been several outbreaks of tuberculosis with multiple drug resistance (MDR) in the USA and Europe including the UK. Transmission of drug-resistant strains has occurred between patients and from patients to family members, health care workers, and prison guards. Mortality from drug-resistant tuberculosis in this setting is high, around 70–90%. To reduce the risk of MDR TB, it is essential to ensure adherence to antituberculosis therapy by patients and for health care facilities to have in place procedures and facilities to reduce the risk of nosocomial transmission.

Treatment of MAC

Clarithromycin 1–2 g/day in divided doses
+
Ethambutol 15 mg/kg/day daily
+
either rifabutin 450–600 mg/day
or rifampicin 450–600 mg/day
and/or ciprofloxacin 500 mg twice daily

3 or 4 drug regimens are recommended

Disseminated infection with *Mycobacterium avium* complex (MAC) causes considerable morbidity and mortality in the later stages of HIV infection (when CD4 counts are persistently $<50 \times 10^6/l$). Various combinations of drugs have been shown to decrease mycobacteraemia and improve symptoms in uncontrolled studies. Four, three, and two drug regimens have and are being assessed in clinical trials. Studies of monotherapy have shown both clinical and microbiological improvement in the short term but relapse occurs and resistance develops frequently. A commonly used regimen in clinical practice is rifampicin or rifabutin (450–600 mg/day), ethambutol (15 mg/kg, max 1 g/day) and clarithromycin (500 mg twice a day). Other drugs that have been studied and may be considered include: ciprofloxacillin (500–750 mg twice a day), parenteral amikacin (7·5–15 mg daily for 2–4 weeks), and another macrolide, azithromycin. Treatment is usually continued for life.

A randomised placebo controlled study of rifabutin 300 mg/day (as primary prophylaxis) in over 500 patients with AIDS and CD4 cell counts $<200 \times 10^6/l$ has shown that there is significantly longer time to MAC bacteraemia and a longer period free of disease. Recent studies also show that clarithromycin (500 mg twice daily) and azithromycin (1200 mg once per week) also reduce the incidence of MAC bacteriaemia and their efficacy may be greater than rifabutin. Emergence of resistant strains on clarithromycin and azithromycin prophylaxis occurs in those who develop bacteraemia and there is cross resistance.

Salmonella spp. infections are treated with either cotrimoxazole or ciprofloxacin and *Campylobacter* spp. with ciprofloxacin. In salmonella infections relapses of enteritis or bacteraemia are common.

Antiviral therapy

The ideal antiviral agent should be specific, orally absorbed, and cross the blood–brain barrier. It should also be free from adverse effects, since the best we can expect is suppression of viral replication; the problem of latently infected cells will remain. Theoretically, inhibition of productive viral replication may allow some recovery of immune function, perhaps encouraging regression of tumours and elimination of the conditions favouring opportunistic infections.

Various potential targets for antiviral treatment have been identified since we have gained a better understanding of the replicative cycle and molecular biology of HIV. The first drugs made available for clinical use were inhibitors of the HIV reverse transcriptase enzyme. Before the virus can be integrated into the host cell's genome, a DNA copy of the viral RNA has to be formed (proviral DNA). This is regulated by the specific HIV DNA polymerase: reverse transcriptase (RT). If a DNA copy is not formed the viral RNA genome becomes susceptible to destruction by cellular enzymes. RT inhibitors include nucleoside analogues that inhibit by chain termination and competitive inhibition of the enzyme and non-nucleoside agents which bind directly to RT and are non-competitive inhibitors.

The ideal antiviral agent—a tall order

- Protects uninfected cells
- Reduces viral production from infected cells
- Specific
- Orally absorbed
- Crosses blood–brain barrier
- No side effects

More recently specific competitive inhibitors of the HIV protease enzyme have been evaluated and are being introduced into clinical use. Inhibition leads to a defective and immature virus particle production by preventing the cleavage of a precursor core protein into several components which the virus requires.

Inhibitors of the HIV integrase enzyme have also been developed and are now undergoing phase I/II clinical trials. HIV replication from its integrated site is controlled by a number of regulatory genes. The *tat* (transactivating transcription) gene codes for a protein that transactivates the promoter in the HIV long terminal repeat (LTR) region which amplifies viral transcription. Clinical trials of *tat* inhibitors have to date been disappointing.

Interferons have a broad spectrum of antiviral activity and act at a number of different sites of viral replication. Alpha interferons have been assessed in combination with other nucleoside analogues, particularly zidovudine but haematological toxicity has been a problem.

Combination therapy

Clinical trials of zidovudine as monotherapy showed that it reduced mortality and the risk of clinical progression in the short term in patients with symptomatic disease, but when used earlier in patients with asymptomatic infection, any clinical benefit was transient and there was no improvement in survival. In addition, zidovudine-resistant HIV strains can be isolated from symptomatic patients receiving more than six months therapy and this resistance is associated with multiple mutations of the reverse transcriptase gene. With these problems of limited clinical efficacy, reduced viral sensitivity over time, and also drug intolerance, combinations of the two or more agents have been investigated and continue to be evaluated in clinical trials.

The aims of combination chemotherapy are to maintain or enhance efficacy through synergy, to use lower doses of drugs with non-overlapping toxicity profiles and to delay the emergence of resistance either by delaying mutations of the RT gene or indeed by conferring multiple mutations which may lead to reversal of resistance or perhaps incompetent virus production (convergent combination chemotherapy).

A combination of zidovudine and didanosine, or zidovudine and zalcitabine has been shown in large clinical trials to improve survival and reduce the rate of progression to AIDS by approximately 40% compared to zidovudine monotherapy over 3 years.

Triple and quadruple combinations including both reverse transcriptase and protease inhibitors are being assessed in clinical trials. Initial results suggest more marked falls in plasma HIV RNA levels, and increases in CD4 count are achieved in the short-term compared to either mono or dual RT inhibitor combination regimens, and evidence of clinical efficacy is emerging (see below).

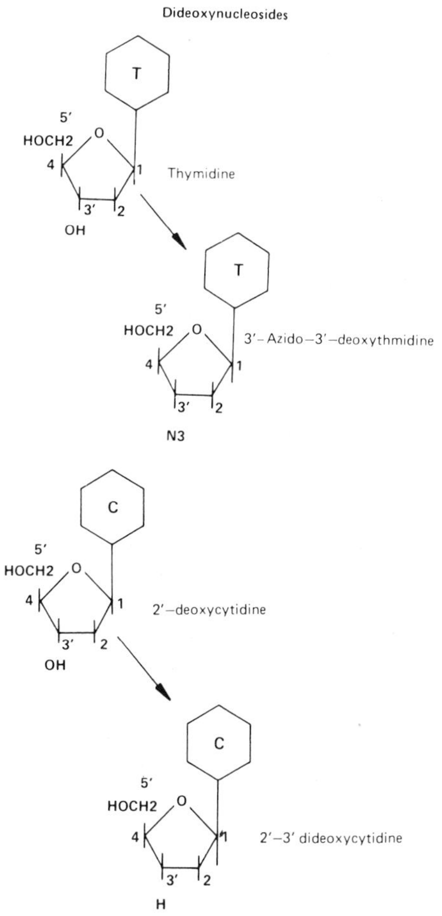

Targets for antiviral therapy

Target	*Treatment*
Virus receptor	Blocking antibodies or ligands
Uncoating of virus	Amantadine-like compounds
Reverse transcriptase	Inhibitors/DNA chain terminators
RNAase	Inhibitors
Integration	Viral "integrase" inhibitors
Viral gene expression	Inhibitors of HIV regulator genes and their products
Viral protein synthesis and assembly	Enzyme inhibitors (for example, viral protease inhibitors)
Viral budding	Interferons (also act at other sites of replication cycle), antibodies, and ligands

Dideoxynucleosides

T
5′
HOCH2
O
4
1
3′
2
OH
Thymidine

T
5′
HOCH2
O
4
1
3′
2
N3
3′–Azido–3′–deoxythmidine

C
5′
HOCH2
O
4
1
3′
2
OH
2′–deoxycytidine

C
5′
HOCH2
O
4
1
3′
2
H
2′–3′ dideoxycytidine

Deoxynucleosides.

Nucleoside analogue inhibitors of reverse transcriptase

The nucleoside analogues are both competitive inhibitors of RT and DNA chain terminators. The normal 2′ deoxynucleosides which are substrates for DNA synthesis link to form a chain by phosphodiester linkages bridging the 5′ and 3′ positions on the five carbon sugar molecule. The 2′, 3′ dideoxynucleosides analogues are formed by the replacement of the 3′ hydroxy group by an azido, hydrogen or other group. The HIV RT enzyme will add these nucleoside analogues to a growing HIV proviral DNA chain. Once inserted, the normal 5′ to 3′ links will not occur resulting in HIV proviral DNA chain termination.

The first of the generation of nucleoside analogues to be evaluated was zidovudine (formerly azidothymidine, AZT). The clinical efficacy of zidovudine has since been demonstrated in combination regimens with didanosine zalcitabine, and lamivudine. The commonest toxicity is bone marrow suppression and this is more severe in patients with advanced disease. Other adverse events include gastrointestinal intolerance particularly in the first few weeks of therapy and myopathy with long-term zidovudine treatment. Multiple mutations of the RT gene have been identified from HIV strains isolated from patients receiving long-term therapy. These mutations are associated with the loss of phenotypic sensitivity to zidovudine.

The main toxicities of didanosine (ddI) are pancreatitis, hepatitis, and peripheral neuropathy, all of which tend to occur more frequently at higher dose and in patients with more advanced disease. It also causes diarrhoea but this is probably related to the buffer in the tablet which needs to be taken on an empty stomach.

Clinical efficacy data support the use of didanosine in combination with zidovudine for initiation of therapy and adding it, or switching to it, in patients taking zidovudine monotherapy. Mutations of the RT gene associated with resistance to didanosine do occur but these develop at a slower rate and are fewer in number than those seen with zidovudine. Combination therapy with didanosine and zidovudine results in a delay in the onset of resistance to didanosine but not to zidovudine.

Anti-retroviral drug treatments for HIV infection

Drugs	*Dose*	*Adverse events*
Reverse transcriptase inhibitors		
Zidovudine	500–600 mg/day in divided doses	Anaemia, neutropenia, gastrointestinal intolerance, myopathy
Didanosine	200 mg twice daily	Diarrhoea, pancreatitis, dry mouth
Zalcitabine	0·75 mg three time daily	Peripheral neuropathy, mouth ulcers
Lamivudine	150 mg twice daily	Few side effects: neutropenia, peripheral neuropathy reported
Stavudine	20–40 mg twice daily	Peripheral neuropathy
Protease inhibitors		
Saquinavir	600 mg three times daily	No serious adverse events. Few reported side effects
Ritonavir	600 mg twice daily	Gastrointestinal tolerance first 2–4 weeks. Abnormal liver function tests. Major drug interactions
Indinavir	800 mg three times daily	Nephrolithiasis, asymptomatic hyperbilirubinemia

Zalcitabine (ddC) is a cytidine analogue and has proven clinical efficacy in combination with zidovudine. However, in patients who have taken zidovudine long term the addition of zalcitabine therapy does not appear to improve clinical outcome further. The side effects of zalcitabine include mouth ulcers and a painful but usually reversible peripheral neuropathy which is dose related and more common than that occurring with didanosine. A limited number of mutations of the RT enzyme have been identified with zalcitabine but they appear infrequently in patients on therapy and their clinical relevance is uncertain. Cross-resistance between didanosine and zalcitabine can occur.

Two other nucleoside analogues are available for clinical use; stavudine (D4T) a thymidine analogue and lamivudine (3TC), another cytidine analogue. Both produce similar changes in plasma HIV RNA levels and rises in CD4 count to that seen with zidovudine monotherapy. In combination with other RT inhibitors greater changes in these surrogate markers have been demonstrated with both drugs. Lamivudine is well tolerated and has few side effects. The main toxicity of stavudine is a peripheral neuropathy. Resistant mutations to lamivudine emerge quickly within a few weeks of therapy but virus populations with this mutation remain sensitive to zidovudine. Resistance to zidovudine may be delayed and, if present, reversed by lamivudine in combination. There are now clinical efficacy data to support the addition of lamivudine in patients either on zidovudine alone, or zidovudine combination with didanosine or zalcitabine.

Non-nucleoside inhibitors of the reverse transcriptase

A group of structurally diverse non-nucleoside RT inhibitors which block enzyme activity through alosteric inhibition has been developed. A number of these show high activity *in vitro* and low toxicity. They are also highly specific, inhibiting the reverse transcriptase of HIV-1 but not HIV-2. However, phase I/II studies have revealed the rapid emergence of resistant strains associated with single point mutations of the RT gene and loss of antiviral effects at the doses used. Despite this these drugs are still likely to be useful in combination therapy and the two most promising, nevirapine and delavirdine are being evaluated as part of combination regimens in large phase III trials.

Protease inhibitors

Protease inhibitors are a new class of specific anti-HIV drugs that have recently been introduced into clinical practice. They bind competitively to the substrate site of the viral protease enzyme which is responsible for the cleavage of a large structural core protein during budding from the infected cell. Inhibition results in a production of immature virus particles.

The development from phase I/II trials to licensing has been rapid and in 1996 three, saquinavir, ritonavir, and indinavir, are available to clinicians for treatment of HIV infection; others are in development. Saquinavir, the first to enter the clinical trials, has poor bioavailability. In combination with zidovudine and zalcitabine, it produces greater falls in plasma HIV RNA levels and increases in CD4 counts than either monotherapy or the zidovudine/zalcitabine combination. There are now clinical efficacy data to support its use in combination therapy. Reported side effects are few; a new formulation is being developed to increase plasma levels.

Ritonavir and indinavir monotherapy produce more pronounced short-term effects on plasma HIV RNA levels and CD4 count, than monotherapy with either standard doses of saquinavir or the currently licensed RT inhibitors. However, a trial of high dose saquinavir monotherapy (7·2 g/day) produces similar changes in plasma RNA levels to indinavir or ritonavir monotherapy at standard doses. The addition of ritonavir to current treatment regimens in patients with CD4 counts $<100 \times 10^6$/l has been shown to reduce mortality and the incidence of further AIDS defining illnesses over six months. Triple combination therapy with indinavir, didanosine and zidovudine has a much greater effect on viraemia and CD4 counts than indinavir monotherapy or the zidovudine/didanosine combination. Multiple mutations in the protease enzyme gene can occur under the selective pressure of therapy with each of the protease inhibitors and result in phenotypic resistance. Common mutations have been identified and cross-resistance can occur. The clinical implications of this have not yet been determined.

Reduction of morbidity in symptomatic disease by:

- Education of physicians and patients
- Improved diagnostic methods
- Earlier diagnosis and treatment of complications
- Improved and alternative treatments for opportunistic infections
- Primary and secondary prophylaxis for *Pneumocystis carinii* pneumonia
- Chronic suppressive therapy for herpes simplex viruses and fungal infections
- Antiviral therapy

Conclusion

The reduction in morbidity and mortality in patients with symptomatic HIV disease documented in observational studies is probably due to many factors: these include increased patient and physician education, improved diagnostic methods leading to earlier diagnosis and treatment, primary and secondary prophylaxis for *Pneumocystis carinii* pneumonia, chronic suppressive therapy for herpes virus and fungal infections as well as improved treatments for the opportunistic infections. In this setting we have also seen the introduction into clinical practice of combination therapy with proven efficacy in terms of morbidity and mortality for up to three years. It is hoped that more potent combinations will further enhance this benefit without it being offset by longer term safety issues.

The clinical efficacy of combination therapy has been demonstrated across a wide range of clinical stages and CD4 strata. The optimal time to start therapy remains uncertain. Clinical practice across Europe and North America varies but most clinicians would consider initiating therapy at some point between a CD4 count of 200 and 500×10^6/l and in all patients who are symptomatic. Apart from drug intolerance, indications to change therapy have not yet been defined and fully evaluated but physicians will use evidence of clinical progression, a falling CD4 count and/or rising plasma RNA levels back towards the level at start of therapy. Analysis of large phase III clinical trials has shown that in addition to baseline CD4 cell count the baseline plasma HIV RNA level and the short-term change in plasma HIV RNA on therapy are independent predictors of clinical outcome. In routine clinical practice the best strategy for monitoring therapy may eventually include CD4 count, plasma HIV RNA levels and genotypic resistance analysis, but further information on how best to use these markers is needed.

The authors wish to thank the Department of Medical Photography and Illustration, the Middlesex Hospital, for the clinical photographs.

10 HIV INFECTION AND AIDS IN THE DEVELOPING WORLD

Kevin M De Cock

Epidemiology of HIV-1 and HIV-2 infections in developing countries

Two distinct viruses causing AIDS, HIV types 1 and 2 (HIV-1/HIV-2), are in worldwide circulation. HIV-1 is responsible for most infections, HIV-2 being very rare outside of West Africa. Individual cases of HIV-2 infection have been described in other parts of Africa, Europe, the Americas, and Asia (India), but most infected persons have had some epidemiologic link to West Africa.

The routes of transmission of HIV-1 and HIV-2 have been described earlier. The transmission of HIV-2 infection is less efficient than that of HIV-1; this applies particularly to perinatal transmission, only about 1% of HIV-2-infected mothers passing the infection on to their offspring; sexual transmission is also less efficient, especially before the development of end-stage immune deficiency. Postnatal transmission of HIV-1 by breast milk is more important than previously believed and may contribute an additional 10–15% to the HIV-1 perinatal transmission rate, with obvious implications for child health in developing countries.

While the routes of HIV-1 and HIV-2 transmission are the same all over the world, the relative importance of different modes of transmission differs in different regions. In most developing countries, heterosexual transmission is the dominant mode of spread, and perinatally acquired HIV infection is therefore much more prevalent than in industrialised countries. Homosexual transmission is rare in Africa, but is more important in south-east Asia and Latin America. Transmission associated with injecting drug use is particularly frequent in parts of south and south-east Asia and Latin America. Acquisition of infection from contaminated blood remains a problem, especially in parts of sub-Saharan Africa and south Asia; in some countries commercial blood donation acts to amplify the spread of transfusion-transmitted HIV infection, both to the recipients of blood as well as to donors who may become infected through exposure to unsterile equipment. Women and children are at especially high risk for transfusion-transmitted HIV infection, the former because of the high incidence of anaemia and haemorrhage associated with pregnancy and childbirth, and the latter because of malarial anaemia.

Natural history of HIV-1 and HIV-2 infections in developing countries

Surprisingly little information is available on the natural history of HIV-1 and HIV-2 infections in the developing world. Evidence from prospective studies in industrialised countries suggests that after 10 years of infection with HIV-1, approximately 50% of persons have AIDS. There is a widespread belief that the natural history in developing countries is more rapid, but evidence to substantiate faster progression of immune deficiency is lacking. Because certain bacterial infections (for example, pneumococcal infection, tuberculosis) may occur at relatively high CD4+ lymphocyte counts, some HIV-infected persons may appear to become symptomatic earlier, and in addition, outcome may be worse in developing countries than in the industrialised world because of lack of access to care. This latter reason is almost certainly largely responsible for the reduced survival following the development of an AIDS-defining illness in developing countries, generally of the order of six to nine months.

The course of HIV-2 infection seems longer than that of infection with HIV-1. Evidence to suggest this includes individual reports of long survival with HIV-2 infection, higher levels of CD4+ lymphocyte counts in HIV-2- than in HIV-1-infected persons in cross-sectional studies, and a lower incidence of CD4+ lymphocyte decline and AIDS in prospective studies of HIV-1- and HIV-2-infected persons. However, considerable overlap can exist in the incubation periods for disease, and the pathogenicity of HIV-2 should not be forgotten.

AIDS

WHO AIDS case definition for AIDS surveillance

For the purposes of AIDS surveillance an adult or adolescent (>12 years of age) is considered to have AIDS if at least two of the following major signs are present in combination with at least one of the minor signs listed below, and if these signs are not known to be due to a condition unrelated to HIV infection.

- *Major signs*
  - weight loss ⩾10% of body weight
  - chronic diarrhoea for >1 month
  - prolonged fever for >1 month (intermittent or constant)
- *Minor signs*
  - persistent cough for >1 month[a, b]
  - generalised pruritic dermatitis
  - history of herpes zoster[b]
  - oropharyngeal candidiasis
  - chronic progressive or disseminated herpes simplex infection
  - generalised lymphadenopathy

The presence of either generalised Kaposi's sarcoma or cryptococcal meningitis is sufficient for the diagnosis of AIDS for surveillance purposes.

[a] For patients with tuberculosis, persistent cough for >1 month should not be considered as a minor sign.
[a, b] Indicates changes from the 1985 provision WHO clinical case definition for AIDS ("Bangui definition").

Box 1

Expanded WHO case definition for AIDS surveillance

For the purposes of AIDS surveillance an adult or adolescent (>12 years of age) is considered to have AIDS if a test for HIV antibody gives a positive result, and one or more of the following conditions are present:

- ⩾10% Body weight loss or cachexia, with diarrhoea or fever, or both, intermittent or constant, for at least 1 month, not known to be due to a condition unrelated to HIV infection
- Cryptococcal meningitis
- Pulmonary or extrapulmonary tuberculosis
- Kaposi's sarcoma
- Neurological impairment that is sufficient to prevent independent daily activities, not known to be due to a condition unrelated to HIV infection (for example, trauma or cerebrovascular accident)
- Candidiasis of the oesophagus (which may be presumptively diagnosed based on the presence of oral candidiasis accompanied by dysphagia)
- Clinically diagnosed life-threatening or recurrent episodes of pneumonia, with or without aetiological confirmation
- Invasive cervical cancer

Box 2

The Centers for Disease Control (CDC) AIDS surveillance case definition, internationally used as a reference, is inapplicable in most developing countries because its use requires access to sophisticated medical investigations. For this reason, the World Health Organisation (WHO) introduced a clinical case definition that could be used under field conditions (Box 1). This definition has recently been expanded to incorporate HIV serology (thus increasing specificity) and to take account of the revisions of the CDC case definition that occurred in the industrialised world (Box 2). In countries where serologic testing is unavailable or inaccessible, the clinical case definition should be used. It should be noted that these developing country definitions were introduced for epidemiologic surveillance and not for clinical care or staging of patients.

Clinical features and disease associations

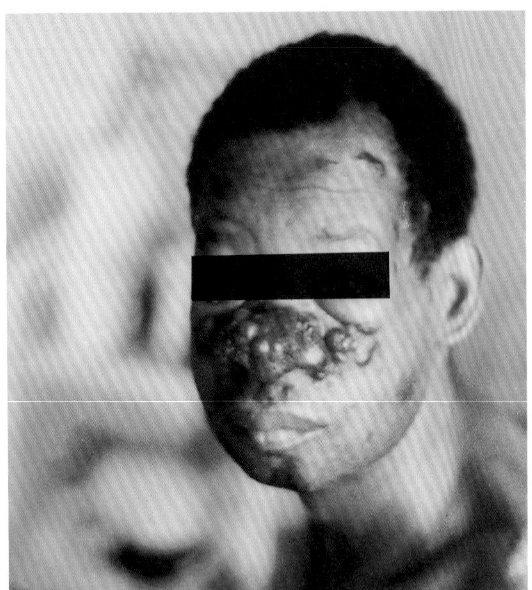

Aggressive Kaposi's sarcoma in a patient with HIV-1 infection.

As in industrialised countries, the spectrum of clinical manifestations associated with HIV infection is wide, ranging from an asymptomatic state to fatal illness owing to opportunistic infections, malignancies, neurologic disease, and wasting. Initial acquisition of HIV infection ("acute HIV infection", or "seroconversion illness") may be complicated by a mononucleosis-like syndrome, sometimes associated with acute meningoencephalitis.

Common symptoms and signs accompanying progressive decline of the level of CD4+ T-lymphocytes, the hallmark of HIV-induced immunodeficiency, are weight loss, fever, night sweats, and diarrhoea. Skin disorders are frequent early manifestations, especially varicella zoster and pruriginous dermatitis, an itchy, papular rash that with scratching leaves pigmented macules.

Tuberculosis is unquestionably the most important opportunistic infection complicating HIV infection in developing countries, and may present early or late in the course of immunodeficiency. When found early in the course of HIV disease, pulmonary tuberculosis is similar to that found in HIV-negative persons. In advanced immunodeficiency, tuberculosis is usually disseminated and multibacillary in nature. Nocardiosis, while much less common, is a differential diagnosis in some areas.

An inadequately recognised manifestation of HIV disease in developing countries has been bacterial septicaemia. Gram negative organisms are found most frequently, especially non-typhoidal *Salmonella* spp. Invasive pneumococcal disease is also frequent, tending to occur earlier than Gram negative infections. In a minority of patients mycobacteraemia is present; this will usually be due to *Mycobacterium tuberculosis* rather than *Mycobacterium avium intracellulare* complex.

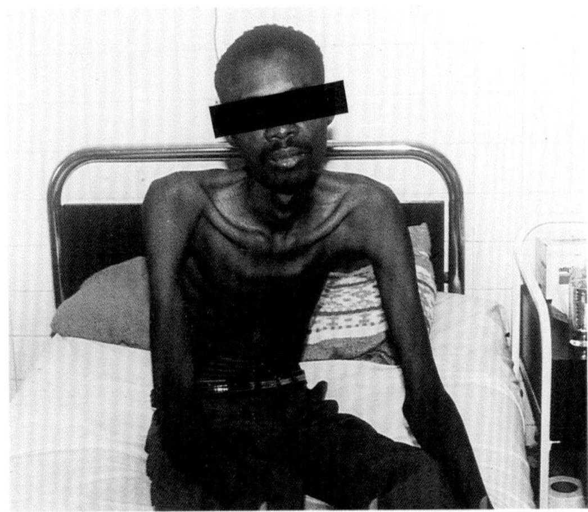

Profound wasting in a patient with a history of weight loss and chronic diarrhoea ("slim disease").

The best known clinical picture of AIDS in Africa is "slim", the term given by persons in rural Uganda to the HIV wasting syndrome. Profound wasting, chronic diarrhoea, and fever are the dominant features. About half the time no specific aetiology can be found for the diarrhoea, although in some cases cryptosporidiosis, microsporidiosis, or isosporiasis are responsible. The commonest autopsy finding in African patients with the HIV wasting syndrome is disseminated tuberculosis, and undue emphasis may have been put on searching for a primary gastrointestinal cause of this whole syndrome. As with all medical causes of wasting, an important contributing factor to the HIV wasting syndrome is reduced food intake.

Cerebral toxoplasmosis and cryptococcal meningitis are probably more frequent in African than Western patients with AIDS. The former most often presents as a space-occupying lesion of the brain, and the latter as a chronic meningitis. Considerable regional variation exists in the frequency of some AIDS-indicator diseases including Kaposi's sarcoma, histoplasmosis, and probably cryptococcosis. Endemic Kaposi's sarcoma is more common in Central and East than in West Africa, and this is probably also true for the AIDS-associated form.

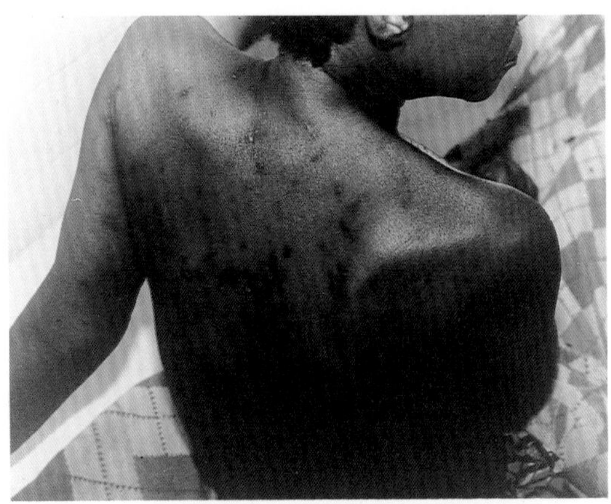

Pruriginous dermatitis in an HIV infected woman. The patient also reported more the 10% loss of body weight.

In south-east Asia, infection with *Penicillium marneffei*, a fungus, results in disseminated disease in advanced immune deficiency, with nodular skin lesions as the most obvious manifestation. Tuberculosis and cryptococcosis are other frequent AIDS-defining conditions in south and south-east Asia. Tuberculosis is frequent in Latin America, where the spectrum of disease is otherwise somewhat more reminiscent of that in the industrialised world.

Certain diseases common in Western patients are rare in AIDS patients in developing countries, including systemic cytomegalovirus disease, pneumocystosis, and infection with atypical mycobacteria such as *Mycobacterium avium intracellulare*. The reasons for this are uncertain, but may include development of diseases such as tuberculosis at higher levels of CD4+ T lymphocyte counts, and inadequate survival with profound immunodeficiency for these other conditions to develop. Some infections present in the tropical environment might be expected to be frequent in HIV disease and are not, such as amoebiasis and strongyloidiasis.

The association between endemic tropical diseases and HIV infection has only been studied to a limited degree. Theoretically, HIV infection could increase the incidence of tropical conditions, and alter their natural history, clinical expression, or response to treatment. Malaria is indirectly linked to HIV infection by causing anaemia in children, who may then be at risk for HIV infection transmitted through blood transfusion. From studies based on limited observations, trypanosomiasis and leprosy do not seem to behave as opportunistic infections, and no information is available concerning the influence of HIV infection on schistosomiasis and filariasis. Visceral leishmaniasis, often with markedly disseminated disease, does appear to be increased in incidence in HIV-infected persons, although most reports have been from southern Europe rather than tropical Africa or South America. Once ill with leishmaniasis, HIV-infected persons require maintenance treatment as relapse is otherwise likely.

Diagnosis

Although advanced AIDS is often easy to diagnose clinically, it is desirable to have HIV serology on patients. The case definitions described in the boxes earlier are intended for epidemiologic surveillance; for clinical purposes a staging system is more useful than a case definition. The table outlines a proposed staging system combining clinical and laboratory data that could be used in developing countries and is currently under evaluation. This system categorises patients into four clinical groups based on clinical features of prognostic significance:

(1) persistent generalised lymphadenopathy;
(2) early (mild) disease;
(3) intermediate (moderate) disease; and
(4) late (severe) disease (essentially similar to AIDS).

A performance scale is also included.

The most useful laboratory marker for clinical staging is the CD4+ T lymphocyte count, although this will rarely be available in developing countries. Absolute levels of lymphocytes can be used as a surrogate, although this is not ideal. Manifestations of HIV disease are rare at CD4+ T lymphocyte counts $>500 \times 10^6$/l and severe illness and death are rare in patients with counts $>200 \times 10^6$/l. Tuberculosis and pneumococcal infection are unpredictable, and may appear at higher as well as lower CD4 T lymphocyte counts. Once patients in developing countries have developed AIDS, they probably die at higher CD4+ T lymphocyte levels than in industrialised countries because of lack of access to high quality medical care; most patients, however, are still dying with advanced immunodeficiency.

Proposed WHO staging system for HIV infection and disease

Patients with HIV infection who are aged ≥13 years are clinically staged on the basis of the presence of the clinical condition, or performance score, belonging to the highest level

	Laboratory stage (A–C)		Clinical stage of disease* (1–4)			
	Total lymphocytes**	CD4+	Asymptomatic	Early	Intermediate	Late
A	>2000	>500	1A	2A	3A	4A
B	1000–2000	200–500	1B	2B	3B	4B
C	<1000	<200	1C	2C	3C	4C

* Group 1: Asymptomatic or generalised lymphadenopathy; normal activity
Group 2: Early stage disease; weight loss <10% body weight, minor mucocutaneous manifestations, varicella zoster within five years, recurrent upper respiratory infections; symptomatic but normal activity
Group 3: Intermediate stage disease; weight loss >10% body weight, unexplained chronic diarrhoea >1 month, unexplained chronic fever >1 month, oral candidiasis, oral hairy leukoplakia, pulmonary tuberculosis within 1 year, severe bacterial infections;
Group 4: CDC-defined AIDS; bed-ridden >50% of day during previous month

** $\times 10^6$/l

Treatment

The general approach to treatment in developing countries should be no different from that in the industrialised world, but is hampered by lack of resources. Antiviral drugs are rarely used because of cost, and diagnostic methods are mostly inaccessible. As for other diseases in resource-poor countries, treatment is often decided based on very limited information.

Patients should be counselled about HIV infection and prevention of its transmission to others. Specific opportunistic infections should be treated as recommended in standard texts. For some, such as tuberculosis and pneumococcal infection, outcome is usually favourable; toxoplasmosis also often responds well to treatment if diagnosed early. Symptomatic treatment sould be directed towards individual symptoms such as diarrhoea or prurigo.

While prophylaxis against certain opportunistic infections prevalent in developing countries is possible, for example against tuberculosis, operational and financial constraints have severely limited the application of this approach.

Future prospects

The burden of HIV and AIDS will increasingly fall on resource-poor countries, and while the most obvious impact will be greatly increased mortality in young adults, HIV infection threatens to erase the public health advances made in maternal and child health, and in tuberculosis control. Demands for health care will be profoundly influenced by the needs of persons with HIV disease, who rapidly fill hospital beds in areas with high rates of HIV infection.

A cautious estimate is that by the year 2000 the cumulative global total of HIV infections and adult AIDS cases may be 40 million and 10 million, respectively; 90% of these HIV infections and cases of AIDS will be in citizens of developing countries. Approximately 10 million children, mostly in the developing world, will have been orphaned by AIDS.

Cosponsors of the Joint United Nations Programme on HIV/AIDS (UNAIDS)

- UNICEF (United Nations Children's Fund)
- UNDP (United Nations Development Programme)
- UNFPA (United Nations Population Fund)
- UNESCO (United Nations Educational, Scientific and Cultural Organization)
- WHO (World Health Organisation)
- The World Bank

Essentials of programmes for HIV/AIDS

In response to the global epidemic of HIV/AIDS, WHO established what later became the Global Programme on AIDS in 1986; in 1994, this body ceased to exist and was replaced by the Joint United Nations Programme on HIV/AIDS (UNAIDS). The initial response called on countries to undertake emergency action as for an acute epidemic, by establishing programmes to combat AIDS through education and other prevention activities. With time, the broader factors behind the emergence of HIV/AIDS became better understood, as did the full socioeconomic impact of the disease and the need for multisectorial involvement in responding to the epidemic.

The global response is based on fundamental principles but HIV/AIDS prevention and control is implemented, successfully or unsuccessfully, at the local level. Involvement of heavily affected communities and non-governmental organizations has been crucial. Recognised basic requirements of programmes have been respect for human rights and confidentiality of HIV-infected persons, integration of sexually transmitted diseases control into HIV/AIDS prevention activities, provision of services for injecting drug users (including, in some countries, methadone maintenance and needle exchange), and, more recently acknowledged, provision of services for HIV/AIDS care as well as prevention. Because of the close interrelationship between HIV/AIDS and tuberculosis, some countries have integrated tuberculosis and HIV/AIDS control activities; this remains a topic of international debate.

Essential components of HIV/AIDS programmes

- Epidemiologic surveillance for HIV infection and AIDS
- Health education
- Blood safety
- STD control (incorporating education for behaviour change, STD treatment, and condom promotion)
- Treatment and prevention services for injecting drug users
- Care for HIV/AIDS
- Protection of human rights of HIV-infected persons, including respect of confidentiality and protection against discrimination

11 INJECTION DRUG USE-RELATED HIV INFECTION

R P Brettle

A variety of medical problems, both infective and non-infective in nature, is associated with injection drug use (IDU) including a number of blood-borne viruses, such as HIV transmitted via the sharing of injection equipment. The medical care of patients using drugs requires a knowledge of both drug- and infection-associated conditions as well as how to deliver the medical care.

Medical care systems

Problems associated with IDU

- Illegal
- Associated with violent or unpredictable behaviour often as a result of drug excess (for example, alcohol/opiates) or drug withdrawals (for example, opiates or benzodiazepines)
- Expensive
- Crisis-type life style
- Day-night reversal

Few if any of the supportive features associated with the management of other groups with HIV and AIDS are present for drug users and the difficulties of engaging drug users for medical care should not be underestimated. IDU has a number of characteristics which are problematic for any health service and increase the difficulty of delivering medical care. These numerous crises whether social, financial, legal etc., lead to the impression of a chaotic life style and hospital appointments have low priority compared to everything else.

The consequences of IDU-related HIV for the individual are also important to recognise since they impact on medical care and carers.

Consequences of drug use related HIV for a Health Service

- Loss of illegal income as a result of both physical and/or mental deterioration
- Increased requests for substitute drugs
- Increased theft in and around hospital premises
- Drug dealing in hospitals settings
- Requests for help in making fraudulent benefit claims
- Inappropriate hospitalisation to save on living expenses

There are a number of additional problems that drug users may suffer from, such as victimisation, harassment, and exploitation. Increasing family anxiety, frequent hospital admissions and self-discharges, increasing use of illegal drugs and harassment often herald the onset of serious HIV encephalopathy or frank dementia which may be missed by professionals. IDU-related admissions to hospital are often complicated by a number of behavioural problems or incidents.

Professionals caring for drugs users also have the added pressures that arise from their peers (nurses, doctors, etc.) who frequently express their displeasure over drug users. Health service staff are naturally alarmed by the prospect of confronting drug users carrying offensive weapons (knives and even on rare occasions guns) although it is often not appreciated that such weapons are for their peers rather than for the staff. The management of drug-using patients also necessitates managing the problem of their visitors.

Problems of IDU in health care settings

- Unexplained absences from wards
- Disruptive visitors
- Self discharges and re-attendance
- Self-medication
- Drug dealing
- Day-night reversal
- Theft
- Noise
- Carrying of offensive weapons

Thus a modified health care system which understands and considers these problems is important. The aim of an IDU service should be to initiate and maintain contact primarily in order to deliver health care and health education. The initiation and maintenance of that contact may require a variety of initiatives.

Initiatives for initiation and maintenance of contact with drug users

- Needle exchange
- Methadone prescribing
- Social provisions such as help with housing
- Medical care

A system of providing both drug services as well as medical care from the same site by the same doctors seems to be an efficient model of care for drug users. Units coping with IDU-related HIV have a number of additional problems that are not usually experienced by other areas of health care.

Specific problems of IDU-related HIV for a Health Service

- Mixture of physical and psychological dependency
- Frequent security and fire incidents
- Increased need for cubicles
- Need for increased staffing levels to cope with cubicles and behaviour

Management strategies for IDU-related HIV

Management strategies for IDU-related admissions

- Continuity of care by medical and nursing staff
- Increased numbers of nursing and medical staff
- Response to violence is to call police
- Tight control on drug prescribing
- A written smoking policy which is given to every patient on admission
- Coordination of drug prescribing between different agencies around admissions and discharges
- Increased contact with health care system gradually
- Clear guidlines and policies which all staff sign up to
- Such policies to be supportive and caring and based on health and safety principles
- Avoid situations leading to confrontation
- Avoid withdrawals in ward area but make it clear that no guarantee of increases on discharge
- Awareness of need for relief of pain and psychological distress

In order to cope with IDU-related HIV admissions it is necessary to consider higher staffing levels, avoidance of high occupancy levels and continuity of care by both nursing and medical staff.

Management of IDU-related problems

Problems of antiretroviral therapy for IDU-related HIV

- Venous access—external jugular in the head-down tilt position preferred
- Possibility of interactions with recreational drugs such as cocaine
- Compliance—12-hour regimes preferred
- Drug interactions
  - opiates double zidovudine levels
  - rifampicin reduces opiate levels
  - protease inhibitors increase opiate and benzodiazepine levels
- Knowledge of controlled drug prescribing

Antiretroviral therapy

The widespread experience with zidovudine suggests that it is perfectly possible to treat current drug users with antiretroviral therapy although there are a number of difficulties in patients requiring monitoring of therapy. Continued IDU does and will occur in patients on antiretroviral therapy and emphasises the importance of continuing with harm reduction messages.

Drug interactions

Little work has been done on interactions of recreational drugs with therapy commonly used in HIV patients. Long-term opiate used doubles zidovudine levels via an interaction at the kidneys. Smaller doses are therefore required to avoid troublesome side effects such as headaches, nausea, and vomiting. No data are available on interactions with other nucleoside analogues. Increased zidovudine levels have also been reported with sodium valproate, a drug that is commonly used to control seizures.

Check list for admission of patients in receipt of addictive drugs

- Amounts and types of drugs regularly prescribed
- Days usually dispensed and date drugs last dispensed from pharmacy
- Check amounts brought into hospital (and amounts therefore "left at home") and record
- Location of various prescriptions
- Suspend or cancel current prescriptions as soon as possible
- Alert general practitioner or prescribing agency of admission
- Alert prescribers if patient allowed out of ward

There are also, of course, a number of important therapeutic drug interactions; for instance, a number of drugs induce hepatic enzymes and established pain control may fail because of lowered opiate drug levels. In drug users this effect may result in severe withdrawal symptoms with concomitant agitation and disruption to the ward area. Common examples include a number of antiepileptics such as phenytoin, and antibiotics such as rifampicin or rifabutin.

Control drug prescriptions

A working knowledge of the regulations surrounding controlled drug prescriptions is important when drug users are being managed. Attention to detail when a patient is admitted is imperative if centres are to avoid the problems of double prescribing. It is important to collect essential information with regard to drug prescriptions.

Medical (non-infection) problems of drug use

Problem	*Medical complications*
Drug effects	
Excess opiate	Narcosis, coma, small pupils, respiratory depression, aspiration pneumonia, and *rhabdomyolysis secondary to pressure*
Opiate withdrawal	Mild "URT" (sweating, coryza, lacrimation), pupillary dilation, insomnia, nausea, vomiting, diarrhoea, lethargy, muscle weakness, myalgia, muscle twitching, tachycardia and hypertension
Excess cocaine	Apprehension, dizziness, syncope, blurred vision, dysphoric states, paranoia, confusion and aggressive behaviour, seizures, coma, hyperthermia, respiratory depression, apnoea, sudden death, spontaneous rhabdomyolysis
Excess amphetamine	Headaches, anorexia, nausea, tremors, dilated pupils, tachycardia, and hypertension
Stimulant withdrawal	Sleepiness, lethargy, increased appetite, food bingeing, depression or even suicide
Trauma	
Frequent injecting	Track marks and skin scars, lack of veins and thrombophlebitis, deep venous thrombosis, persistent peripheral oedema, venous stasis, and ulcers secondary to chronic venous obstruction
Misplaced injections	Arterial damage and insufficiency with secondary tissue damage, muscle compartment syndrome and traumatic rhabdomyolysis, false aneurysms and pulmonary emboli, traumatic neuropathy
Immunology	
IDU	Enlarged nodes, elevated IgM, false positive syphilis serology
Endocrinology	
Opiate use	Increase prolactin levels and gynecomastia, amenorrhoea (may be secondary to weight loss)
Cannabis	Oligospermia, impotence, and gynecomastia
Neurology	
Stimulants	Psychosis, depression, cerebral infarcts, and haemorrhages (CVAs)
Chronic use of benzodiazepines or barbiturates	Brain damage
Cardiology	
Cocaine	Cardiac arrhythmias such as sinus tachycardia, ventricular tachycardia, and fibrillation, as well as asystole, myocardial infarction, severe hypertension
Adulterants of illicit drugs, e.g. quinine	Cardiac arrhythmias and death
Tricyclic antidepressants	Cardiac arrhythmias and death
Cannabis	Sinus tachycardia and postural hypotension
Pulmonary	
Inhaled cocaine	Excessive use of Valsalva—spontaneous pneumomediastinum and pneumopericardium
Excess sedatives or stimulants	Respiratory depression, coma, and pneumonia
Opiate withdrawals	Mild "URT"
Stimulant use such as cocaine	Tachypnoea
Opiates or cocaine	Pulmonary oedema
Hepatitis B	Polyartertis nodosa
Foreign body emboli (particles injected intravenously, for example talc granulomas)	Pulmonary hypertension (and right heart failure), abnormal pulmonary function, such as reduced DCO, restrictive defect due to interstitial lung disease
Smoking of tobacco, heroin, marijuana	Abnormal pulmonary function, such as reduced DCO, COAD
"Snorting" stimulants	Chronic rhinitis, rhinorrhoea, anosmia, atrophy of the mucosal membranes, ulceration, and perforation of the nasal septum
"Snorting" opiates	Recurrent sinusitis

The medical effects of recreational drugs

Those working with drug users also require a working knowledge of the effects of recreational drugs and if necessary the equivalent doses of drugs such as methadone or valium if patients need to be temporarily covered for withdrawals. Tables of equivalence for opiates and benzodiazepines can be found on pages 42 and 45 of the *Guidelines on Clinical Management, Drug Misuse and Dependence*, HMSO. The medical problems associated with IDU are extensive and are summarised here.

Opiates

Management of patients with respiratory infection on opiates

- For mild respiratory depression consider a temporary reduction in oral drugs (10–20%) or splitting the once daily dose into 3 or 4 doses
- When rapid improvement in pulmonary function is required, use naloxone infusions to achieve an acceptable improvement in respiratory rate (and therefore oxygenation) without too great an increase in physical arousal
- Commence a naloxone infusion (2 mg in 500 ml, starting at around 10 ml per hour) which may be required for up to 48 hours in the case of methadone because of its relatively long half life
- If no venous access then use regular small doses of i.m. nalaoxone; 0·2 mg i.m. every hour initially and titrate dose or frequency up or down depending on the response

Excess opiates

The clinical features of excessive doses of opiates are detailed here, and in such patients on maintenance doses of opiates it is always worth considering reversing the effects of opiates even if the patient has taken other sedative drugs such as benzodiazepines. If necessary try a small test dose of naloxone to see whether any improvement in respiration can be achieved. Large doses are best avoided since the resulting disruptive behaviour may result in the loss of venous access. Opiated patients with respiratory problems may require alterations in the dose or actual reversal of opiates.

Opiate withdrawal syndrome

Opiate withdrawals should be considered in any agitated patient particularly those that have recently commenced drugs that induce liver enzymes such as rifampicin, rifabutin, phenytoin, etc. In the latter case increased doses (3–4-fold) will be required.

Stimulants

The excessive use of stimulants such as cocaine can also produce an agitated patient and the distictive features are shown (see Box).

Marijuana/cannabis

Marijuana's effects are primarily psychic, usually euphoria, although it can be associated with confusion, restlessness, emotional lability, pseudohallucinations, anxiety, and toxic psychosis. There is no evidence of a true withdrawal syndrome; sudden withdrawal for a regular user may be associated with hyperirritability, restlessness, and insomnia similar to the withdrawal reaction for alcohol or sedatives.

Benzodiazepines

Excessive *benzodiazepines* produce increasing drowsiness, slurred speech, incoordination, ataxia, and eventually coma. Withdrawal from benzodiazepines may be associated with panic attacks, restlessness, shortness of breath, agitation, and seizures but this may not occur immediately and can last for 6–8 weeks.

Medical problems of HIV-infected drug users

Drug use or HIV?

The extent of IDU-related conditions requires consideration of not only the clinical features of IDU but also the medical conditions associated with HIV since confusion may arise as to the aetiology of specific symptoms. It is therefore important to be aware of the medical problems of HIV as well as those of drug use, particularly injection drug use.

Pre-AIDS deaths

The phenomenon of pre-AIDS death amongst HIV-infected drug users was described soon after the onset of the AIDS epidemic in the USA and accounted for up to 50% of all deaths in drug users; for every AIDS-related death in a drug user, there was one other as a consequence of conditions such as tuberculosis, endocarditis, and bacterial pneumonia. A similar problem was reported from Europe: for instance, in Amsterdam 20% of drug users but only 0·7% of homosexuals died without an AIDS diagnosis. Although pre-AIDS death rates are in part related to excessive drugs the temporal increases over time also suggest a relation with advancing HIV infection. Many overdose deaths in drug users may in fact have a dual pathology, an interaction between the effects of the drugs and the effects of HIV, for instance pneumonitis which might increase the depressant effects of drugs such as opiates.

Examples of conditions caused by both drug use and HIV

- Lymphadenopathy is associated with IDU
- Fatigue, lethargy, and excessive sweating are also caused by mild withdrawal from opiates
- Diarrhoea is also a common symptom of opiate withdrawal
- Weight loss and fever are both associated with heavy opiate or stimulant (amphetamines or cocaine) use
- Epileptic seizures occur with the intermittent use of benzodiazepines or in hepatic encephalopathy
- The excessive use of cannabis and benzodiazepines or frequent head injuries interfere with memory
- Syncopal attacks are associated with tricyclic antidepressants such as amitriptylene
- Jaundice may occur as a result of acute or chronic hepatitis B or C infection
- Shortness of breath and a persistent cough can occur with endocarditis, bacterial pneumonia, excessive smoking, recurrent bronchitis and obstructive airways disease

Respiratory infections

The annual incidence of bacterial pneumonia and ensuing death is increased in HIV positive drug users compared both to non-drug-using positives and negatives.

In Edinburgh the commonest single identifiable reason for an HIV admission was because of a respiratory tract infection (29% of all admissions) and *Haemophilus influenzae* rather than *Streptococcus pneumonia* was the commonest organism isolated.

Additional susceptibility factors for drug users may include the depressant effect of opiates on the cough reflex as well as the immune system. Recently it has been suggeted that the inhalation of recreational drugs increases the risks of bacterial pneumonias. The odds of developing pneumonia were twice as great for those reporting smoking cocaine, crack cocaine, and marijuana, and increased >20-fold for those also having prior PCP and a low CD4 count.

The incidence of tuberculosis is much higher in HIV-infected drug users, than in other risk groups outside the tropics, or in HIV-negative drug users. In the USA, possibly four times as many patients with AIDS and tuberculosis have been drug users compared to other risk groups.

Hepatitis

Drug users with a history of IDU are likely to have been infected with viruses such as hepatitis B and C. In most series at least 80% have markers of these viral conditions. Approximately 10% of drug users will be carriers of hepatitis B and reactivation with reappearance of antigen as the immune dysfunction advances is well described. Repeat testing for the presence of HBsAg with the onset of immunodeficiency is therefore required. The effect of hepatitis C on HIV is as yet unknown but may account for many of the liver problems described in drug-using cohorts.

HIV dementia and encephalitis

HIV/AIDS is unusual in that it combines both immunological, neurological, and psychiatric disorders, and as a consequence patients may develop a variety of disabilities ranging from wasting disorders, severe pain, neurological dysfunction, such as paralysis, or cognitive impairment and psychological symptoms. Autopsy studies in Edinburgh have shown that as many as 60% of IDU-related HIV patients have evidence of HIV encephalitis although only 6–7% have frank dementia.

Whilst all risk groups may be affected, management issues are more complex with drug users since the patients may become quite susceptible to the effects of recreational and neuroleptic drugs. They find it difficult to accept that they can no longer tolerate "normal" doses of recreational drugs and the symptoms of cognitive impairment are worsened by benzodiazepines, marijuana, or stimulants as well as intercurrent infections or fever.

An accurate diagnosis is an important aid to a management plan which may be based around behavioural therapy. Considerable supervision of the patient is required to prevent wandering or harm to either the patient or others. This is obviously important in wards where patients with infective conditions are located. The greatest danger for IDU-related HIV dementia is access to illegal drugs from patients or visitors who do not appreciate their sensitivity to such drugs, and the problems of fire from smoking.

AIDS

In drug users, Kaposi's sarcoma, cytomegalovirus and chronic cryptosporidiosis are all significantly less common than for all other risk groups notified with AIDS, while PCP, tuberculosis, oesophageal candidiasis and extrapulmonary cryptococcosis are more common.

Psychological disturbances

Although psychological disturbances may occur in all patients with HIV it is the impression that they are now common in IDU-related HIV. In addition to the usual anxieties over HIV problems, frank psychosis is a very real problem. In many, the underlying cause is drug-related, particularly from stimulants such as amphetamines, cannabis, and the irregular use of benzodiazepines. Problems appear to be commoner in the presence of HIV encephalitis, and management requires an accurate diagnosis including an evaluation for HIV encephalitis.

Progression from HIV to AIDS

Extensive reviews of progression to AIDS in cohorts of various risk groups with known length of infection, revealed rates of progression of 0–2% at two years, 5–10% at four years, 10–25% at six years, 30–40% at eight years and 48% at 10 years. An Italian study of drug users with seroconversion rates estimated that there was a 5% progression rate by year three to four and a 21% progression rate to AIDS after six to seven years of HIV infection. By comparison, in Edinburgh progression rates to AIDS in drug users with known seroconversion dates suggest figures of 6–11% after six to seven years and 31% by 10 years with an estimated mean incubation time to AIDS of 11·6 years. No evidence has been found for a role of alcohol, opiates, or other psychoactive drugs in accelerating the progression of immunodeficiency in HIV-seropositive homosexual and bisexual men. A lower probability of disease progression was noted among methadone users or ex-users compared to those that continued IDU in Switzerland. The major factors identified in progression of HIV appear to be age and HLA type. A1 B8 DR3 and Bw35 are all associated with more rapid progression whilst B27 is associated with slower progression to AIDS and death. The phenomonon of non-progression of HIV has been recognised but the number of individuals not progressing is as yet poorly estimated and depends very much upon the definition employed. Consequently depending upon the study, estimates of anywhere between 2–30% have been suggested.

Survival after the development of AIDS

Without treatment, in general, around 50% of patients with AIDS survive one year but only a fifth for three years and the median survival time is around 18–20 months. In Edinburgh the one- and three-year post-AIDS survival rates were 66% and 25%. Older age at AIDS diagnosis and HLA type A1 B8 DR3 were associated with shorter survival. Whilst it had been generally assumed that the survival for injection drug users with AIDS would be shorter than for other risk groups, several studies including our own counter this presumption.

12 HIV INFECTION IN CHILDREN

Gareth Tudor-Williams, Diana M Gibb

Prevalence of HIV infection and AIDS in children

Over 1·5 million children cumulatively are estimated to have been infected with HIV worldwide. The great majority (>80%) have acquired the virus through mother-to-child transmission with approximately 360 000 new cases being born annually. An increasing proportion of women in Europe and the US are being infected through heterosexual transmission rather than from intravenous drug use (IVDU) or from infected blood/blood products. In many countries screening of blood and blood products and exclusion of high-risk donors have resulted in eradication of infection acquired through this route. However, in some countries such as Romania, the majority of children acquired HIV through infected blood. In the US, and recently in the UK, children and young teenagers are being reported with HIV infection acquired through sexual transmission including sexual abuse.

The prevalence and patterns of HIV infection in children are being monitored in different geographical areas through notifications of paediatric AIDS cases, registers of HIV infected children and unlinked anonymous testing of antenatal and neonatal blood samples. In the European region 6 060 children with AIDS had been reported to the WHO European AIDS Surveillance Centre by the end of 1995. Over half were reported from Romania (3 403), but there were also reports from over 40 countries including Spain (707), France (600), Italy (530) and the UK (215). Excluding Romanian children, 82% were infected through perinatal transmission. In southern Europe, Scotland and Ireland, the majority of mothers are IVDUs whereas in France, Belgium, and England, most mothers have acquired the virus through heterosexual transmission in a high prevalence country, most frequently sub-Saharan Africa.

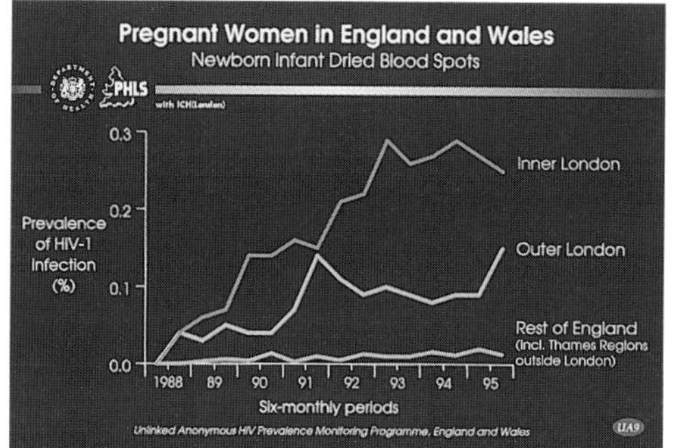

Trends in prevalence of HIV infection in pregnant women by area of residence in England and Wales, from unlinked anonymous monitoring programme using Guthrie cares, 1988–1995. (Courtesy of Public Health Laboratory.)

Unlinked anonymous monitoring of HIV through testing newborn dried blood spot samples (Guthrie cards) is occurring in many countries in Europe and the US and provides an unbiased estimate of the prevalence of HIV infection among pregnant women having live babies. This is being conducted throughout London, and covers 60% of all births in the UK. In 1995 the prevalence of maternal infection was 1:380 in inner London and 1:840 in outer London. The prevalence in Lothian and Tayside in Scotland was 1:1 146. In the rest of the UK outside metropolitan London the prevalence was 1:8 400. The rise in seroprevalence has been most significant in inner London. The majority of known HIV-infected children also live in London; as of April 1996, 276 of the total 389 vertically HIV-infected children reported to the combined Obstetric and Paediatric confidential registers covering the UK and Irish Republic were from London, and 80% were born to mothers who had spent time in sub-Saharan Africa.

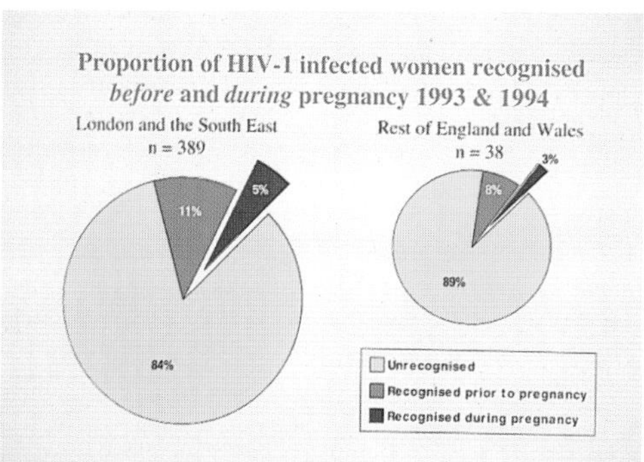

Proportion of HIV-1 infected women in England and Wales recognised before and during pregnancy, 1993–1994.

It is possible to calculate that at the present time only about 10–15% of infected pregnant women in London and the rest of the UK, excluding Scotland, know their HIV status prior to delivery. This was the situation in 1995 as well as in 1993 and 1994. Despite Department of Health guidelines advocating that all women in high prevalence areas are offered HIV testing, uptake of testing in pregnancy is low in London (about 5–60%) and even lower outside London. In other European countries, such as France and Sweden, antenatal HIV testing is offered and accepted by the majority of pregnant women nationwide. Opportunities to reduce transmission of HIV from mothers to their infants are therefore being missed in the UK.

Transmission of HIV infection from mother to child

The risk of transmission from mother to child without intervention varies from about 15–35%. The lowest rates are reported from populations of non-breastfeeding women in Europe (15–20%), the highest (35%) from Africa. Transmission is increasingly thought to occur mainly around the time of delivery, and is influenced by multiple factors. Higher maternal viral load has been shown to be associated with increased transmission, as have factors assumed to reflect viral load including low maternal CD4 + lymphocyte counts and advanced clinical HIV disease. Longer duration of labour, and intervals of >4 hours from membrane rupture to delivery may be associated with higher transmission rates. The mode of delivery may also be important. A meta-analysis of prospective studies showed a modest overall benefit of caesarean section over vaginal delivery, but there are conflicting data with some studies showing no difference in transmission rates attributable to mode of delivery. The morbidity from caesarean section may be higher in HIV infected women compared with uninfected women. At this time, therefore, elective caesarean section cannot be universally advocated for HIV-infected women and a randomised trial to address this has started in Europe and South Africa.

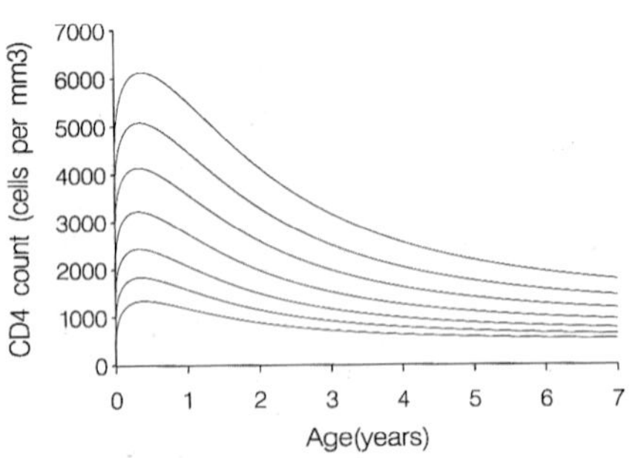

Normal ranges for absolute CD4 + lymphocyte counts in children.

HIV is present in breast milk and a meta-analysis of several prospective studies indicated an additional risk of transmission of 14% among women who breastfeed. Although bottle feeding is recommended for HIV-infected women in developed countries, this would not be appropriate in countries or settings where rates of infectious diseases and poor sanitation are high and where artificial feeding would result in increased infant mortality.

Results of the American/French randomised placebo controlled trial (ACTG 076) of zidovudine (AZT) given to previously untreated women during pregnancy, delivery, and to the neonate for six weeks, resulted in a two-thirds reduction of HIV transmission from 25% in the placebo group to 8% in the treated group. The only short term side effect reported in the infants was mild anaemia which resolved without specific treatment on completion of therapy. Reductions in transmission of this order are now being reported from other centres and countries where AZT is being used in pregnancy. The challenge now is to establish whether antiretroviral combinations could reduce transmission even further and whether the length of treatment can be shortened and which drugs would be preferable for mothers who have already received AZT before pregnancy. Long-term follow-up of all babies exposed to drugs perinatally is required to ensure the absence of possible long-term adverse effects.

Reducing perinatal transmission to below 5% is a realistic goal, and currently most women who know their status refrain from breast feeding and accept advice regarding the use of AZT perinatally. However the 85–90% of women whose status remains unrecognised in pregnancy are likely to breast feed and to have transmission rates around 25–30%.

Diagnosis

IgG antibodies to HIV are passively transferred to virtually all babies born to infected mothers. These persist at detectable levels for up to 18 months, which means that waiting for antibodies to become undetectable ("seroreversion") is a slow way to establish the child's infection status. Using techniques that detect the virus or its components directly (polymerase chain reaction (PCR) or other amplification techniques, virus culture, and immune complex dissociated p24 antigen (ICD p24 antigen), 95% of infected infants can be diagnosed by one month of age. EDTA samples for PCR assays can be sent to a reference laboratory, for example at the Public Health Laboratories at Colindale. Virus culture, however, is a highly specialised assay that is available only in research laboratories. ICD p24 antigen is quantitated by a commercial ELISA kit. This is the least sensitive of the three methods.

Suggested follow-up of infants born to HIV infected mothers

Age	*Test*	*Action/interpretation*
24–48 hours	• PCR • ICD p24 antigen • Virus culture (if available)	If positive, suggests intrauterine transmission or high intrapartum innoculum: may be associated with more rapid disease progression. Not helpful if negative, as <50% of infected babies can be detected within 48 hours of birth. Occasional false positive ICD p24 antigen reported at this age
2–4 weeks	• PCR • ICD p24 antigen • Virus culture (if available)	Should detect 95% of infected infants. A positive result must be confirmed on two separate blood samples.
3 months	• PCR • ICD p24 antigen • Virus culture (if available) • ±HIV IgA	If all assays are negative and there are no clinical concerns, the child is almost certainly uninfected.
12–18 months	HIV antibody test	Performed until seroreversion documented.

PCR: polymerase chain reaction; ICD p24 antigen: immune complex dissociated p24 antigen assay; IgA: immunoglobulin A assay.
Note: in London the current Roche PCR may not pick up divergent African viruses, and alternative amplification techniques such as Nucleic Acid Sequence Based Amplification (NASBA) or the Chiron branched chain DNA assay may be required.

If all three assays are negative at three different time points, with at least one set performed at or after 3 months of age, and provided the maternal virus can be detected by the assay, and there are no clinical concerns, the parents/guardians can be informed that their baby is almost certainly not infected. If virus culture is not available, a fourth negative PCR or HIV-specific immunoglobulin A (IgA) is advisable beyond 3 months of age to establish with reasonable certainty that the child is uninfected. IgA assays are highly specific, but lack sensitivity in the first 3 months of life.

T-cell subsets and measurement of immunoglobulins (Ig) are non-specific tests. Reversal of the CD4:8 ratio and high Ig levels (>2 × upper limit of normal) are suggestive of infection but, for diagnostic purposes, should be supported by at least one other test that detects the virus directly. It is important to realise that absolute CD4 counts are physiologically much higher in infants and young children than in adults (figure, p. 64).

All children presumed to be uninfected should be followed until seroreversion is confirmed.

Clinical manifestations

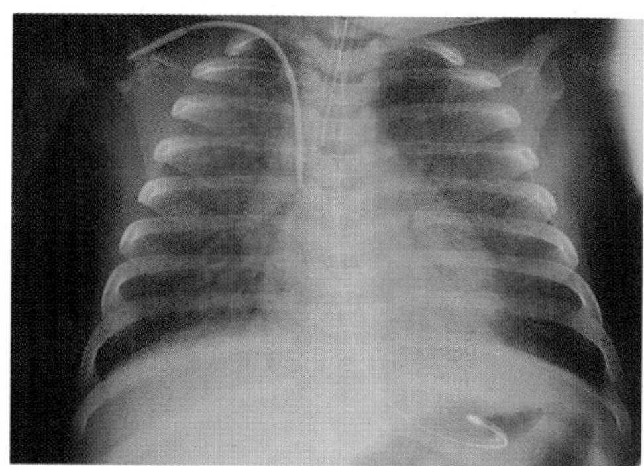

Pneumocystis carinii pneumonia (PCP) in a 3-month-old infant. Diffuse bilateral ground-glass opacificaton, tending to confluence in right upper and both lower lobes. Air bronchograms are seen, which imply air space disease, a late feature of disease. The earliest infiltrates are usually perihilar. The absence of pleural effusion or hilar adenopathy is typical. Less typical presentations include miliary, coin and nodular leisions, lobar consolidation, and cavitations.

As in adults, HIV-infected children present with a spectrum of signs and symptoms reflected in the revised Centers for Disease Control classification system. The differences between adults and children with HIV disease are summarised (table, p. 67). Disease progression is generally faster than in adults with 15–20% of children developing AIDS-defining illnesses by 12 months. This subset of perinatally infected children typically present with *Pneumocystis carinii* pneumonia (PCP) at around 3–4 months of age. Approximately 70% of perinatally infected children will have some signs or symptoms by 12 months. The median age at which children progress to AIDS is about 6 years, and 25–30% have died by this age. The median age of death is around 9 years.

Children with HIV infection frequently present with signs and symptoms that are common in general paediatrics and are non-specific. The most usual clinical features associated with HIV infection include persistent generalised lymphadenopathy, hepatosplenomegaly, chronic or recurrent diarrhoea, fever, and recurrent otitis or sinusitis. Persistent oral candidiasis, parotitis or neurological signs are more specific of HIV infection. Recurrent and often severe bacterial infections are frequent and include pneumonia, cellulitis, local abscesses, osteomyelitis, septic arthritis, and occult bacteraemia. The common causative organisms are

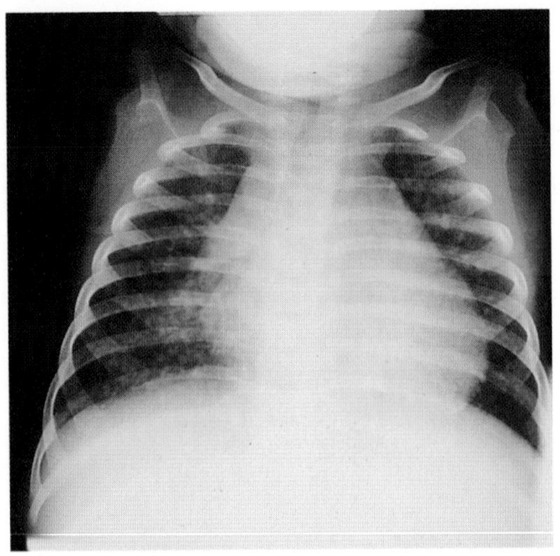

Lymphoid interstitial pneumonitis (LIP) in a child aged 12 months. Diffuse, well-circumscribed nodules distributed uniformly throughout both lung fields. May be associated with hilar adenopathy. A radiological spectrum is seen in LIP, ranging from fine linear interstitial infiltrates to large nodules that tend to confluence in the right middle and lingular lobes.

similar to those seen in children with hypogammaglobulinaemia and include *Pneumococci* spp., *Haemophilus influenzae*, *Staphylococci*, *Streptococci*, and *Salmonellae* spp. This reflects the B cell defect that accompanies the destruction of the CD4-positive helper T-cells. Children with HIV infection frequently have hypergammaglobulinaemia due to dysregulated polyclonal B cell activation. The antibodies are generally nonfunctional.

Pulmonary disease is an important cause of morbidity and mortality and may be one of the first manifestations. Lymphoid interstitial pneumonitis, characterised by multiple foci of proliferating lymphocytes in the lung interstitium, occurs in 20–30% of vertically infected children, but is rare in adults. It presents with persistent bilateral reticulonodular shadowing on chest X-ray and clinical features ranging from asymptomatic to chronic hypoxia. It may be an abnormal response to primary EBV infection.

Centers for Disease Control 1994 revised classification system for HIV infection in children less than 13 years old

- Category N: no symptoms
- Category A: mildly symptomatic
  - lymphadenopathy
  - hepatomegaly
  - splenomegaly
  - dermatitis
  - parotitis
  - recurrent upper respiratory tract infections, sinusitis, or otitis media
- Category B: moderately symptomatic

  Examples of conditions in clinical category B include:
  - anaemia, neutropenia or thrombocytopaenia
  - bacterial infections: pneumonia, bacteraemia (single episode)
  - candidiasis, oropharyngeal
  - cardiomyopathy
  - diarrhoea, recurrent or chronic
  - hepatitis
  - herpes stomatitis, recurrent
  - lymphoid interstitial pneumonia
  - nephropathy
  - persistent fever >1 month
  - varicella (persistent or complicated primary chicken pox or shingles)
- Category C: severely symptomatic

  Any condition listed in the 1987 surveillance case definition for AIDS, with the exception of LIP. For example:
  - serious bacterial infections, multiple or recurrent
  - candidiasis (oesophageal, pulmonary)
  - cytomegalovirus disease with onset of symptoms at age >1 month
  - cryptosporidiosis or isosporiasis with diarrhoea persisting 1 month
  - encephalopathy
  - lymphoma
  - *Mycobacterium tuberculosis*, disseminated or extrapulmonary
  - *Mycobacterium avium* complex or *M. kansasii*, disseminated
  - *Pneumocystis carinii* pneumonia
  - progressive multifocal leukoencephalopathy
  - toxoplasmosis of the brain with onset at age >1 month
  - wasting syndrome

Opportunistic infections, apart from PCP in the subset of children with very rapid disease progression, are usually a late complication of HIV infection and result from severe immunosuppression. The most common are oesophageal candidiasis, multidermatomal varicella zoster, disseminated herpes simplex or cytomegalovirus infections, cryptosporidiosis, and more rarely, toxoplasmosis.

Encephalopathy due to effects of HIV infection on the central nervous system is seen most frequently in the sub-group of children with rapid disease progression. The most common neurological manifestations are spastic diplegia, developmental delay (particularly affecting motor skills and expressive language), or acquired microcephaly. Cranial imaging studies may show basal ganglia calcification and cerebral atrophy and MRI scans may show evidence of white matter damage. Seizures are not a feature of HIV encephalopathy which does not tend to affect the grey matter. The majority of school age children are attending normal school without requiring additional support in the classroom.

Malignancy, such as Kaposi's sarcoma or lymphoma, is a relatively uncommon feature of paediatric HIV disease, accounting for only 1–2% of AIDS-defining illness in children.

Management

For the present time, the aim of any intervention for HIV-infected children should be to maintain the best possible quality of life for the child for as long as possible. This inevitably means balancing the potential benefits of new treatments against the need for increased monitoring and possible toxicities. Management can be considered under four headings: anti-retroviral therapy, prophylactic measures, treatment of opportunistic infections and LIP, and supportive care.

Anti-retroviral therapy

Virus replication in children, as in adults, is occurring at all stages of HIV infection and, as improved drugs and drug combinations become available, treatment is likely to be offered increasingly early. At the present time, however, only the nucleoside analogues such as zidovudine (AZT), dideoxyinosine (ddI) and zalcitabine (ddC) are widely available for children. Clinical trials in children have supported adult studies in demonstrating that AZT monotherapy is less effective than the combination of AZT and ddI. One study has shown ddI monotherapy to be equally effective at delaying disease progression in children as the combination of AZT and ddI. However, AZT penetrates the blood–brain barrier appreciably better than ddI or ddC and should still be included in the treatment of children with overt HIV encephalopathy.

In view of the many uncertainties regarding optimal treatment, it is strongly recommended that children should be offered treatment as part of a clinical trial. Paediatricians in Europe, Brazil, and Canada are collaborating in a series of studies coordinated by the Paediatric European Network for the Treatment of AIDS (PENTA). Combinations of AZT and ddC for treatment naive children, and triple combinations including 3TC for previously treated children are nearing completion. Information about the PENTA studies is available through the Medical Research Council Clinical Trials Centre in London (Tel: 0171 380 9991; Fax: 0171 380 9972) or INSERM in Paris (Tel: 00 33 1 45595201; Fax: 00 33 1 45595180). Protease inhibitors are showing considerable promise as part of combination regimens in adults. Developing palatable formulations for children has been difficult, but nelfinavir in particular appears to be well tolerated and will be assessed in the next PENTA trials enrolling shortly.

Clinical differences between children and adults with HIV disease

- More rapid disease progression
  - 20% of children develop AIDS by 12 months
  - child may be the first family member to present
- Growth faltering is common (affects height and weight)
- Encephalopathy presents with developmental delay and spastic diplegia
- Opportunistic pathogens encountered for the first time
  - primary illnesses often more severe than OIs in adults
- Poor primary responses to childhood infections/immunisations
- Lymphoid interstitial pneumonitis is common
- Malignancy is uncommon

Prophylactic measures

Early onset PCP is a preventable disease. Provided HIV-infected mothers are identified during pregnancy, their infants can be started on PCP prophylaxis from around four weeks of age onwards. Prophylaxis can be stopped once it has been established that the baby is uninfected. Infected children should continue on prophylaxis throughout the first year of life, as CD4 counts are unreliable indicators of risk (see page 64). Thereafter, it is not unreasonable to stop prophylaxis for children with CD4 counts consistently >15%, provided the family are reliable clinical attendees and the child's clinical status and immune function can be regularly monitored. Any child with rapidly declining CD4 counts or counts consistently <15% should be on prophylaxis. Cotrimoxazole is the drug of choice. Regimens vary, but one convenient dosage regime is suggested here. Even with good compliance, PCP breakthrough can occur which may require treatment with alternative agents such as intravenous pentamidine. Rashes and bone marrow suppression due to cotrimoxazole may require the switching to alternative prophylactic agents such as dapsone.

Routine active immunisation schedules should be followed for HIV infected or exposed infants, with the exception that BCG should not be given to symptomatic infected children because of the risk of dissemination. There is a theoretical risk of paralytic poliomyelitis in immunocompromised contacts of children excreting live polio vaccine virus. Inactivated polio vaccine is therefore recommended by injection instead of the live oral polio vaccine. Pneumococcal vaccine is recommended for HIV infected children >2 years of age, and conjugate vaccines may be useful for younger children in the future. Influenza vaccine is generally offered each winter, although data demonstrating its efficacy in this population are lacking.

Suggested doses of cotrimoxazole for prophylaxis for *Pneumocystis carinii* pneumonia

Surface area (m^2)	*Dose of cotrimoxazole* (mg)*
0·25–0·39	240
0·40–0·49	360
0·50–0·75	480
0·76–1·0	720
>1·0	960 (adult dose)

* Dose to be given once daily on three days per week (usually Monday, Wednesday, and Friday). Dose is based on 900 mg/mg^2/dose. Neonates <36 weeks give 450 mg/m^2/dose.

Passive immunisation of symptomatic children is recommended if they are in contact with varicella zoster virus (VZV) and are either VZV naive or have no detectable specific antibodies to VZV. Varicella zoster immunoglobulin (VZIG) ideally should be given within 72 hours of contact. VZIG may prolong the incubation period to 28 days, so clinicians need to consider isolating these patients at clinic visits. Similarly normal human immunoglobulin should be given for susceptible symptomatic children in contact with measles.

Regular intravenous immunoglobulin infusions (400 mg/kg every 28 days) should be reserved for children with recurrent bacterial infections despite good compliance with cotrimoxazole prophylaxis, or for those with proven hypogammaglobulinaemia. Higher doses may be useful in the management of thrombocytopenia (0·5–1·0 g/kg/dose every day, for three to five days).

HIV infected children who are household or day care contacts of individuals with open pulmonary tuberculosis should be carefully assessed, bearing in mind skin testing is frequently unhelpful because of anergy. If there is no evidence of infection, prophylactic isoniazid is recommended. There is little enthusiasm for prophylaxis against *Mycobacterium avium intracellulare* in children because of adverse reactions and the potential for resistance and breakthrough on single agents such as rifabutin.

Treatment of opportunistic infections and LIP

Oropharyngeal candidiasis rarely responds to nystatin in this population, therefore, miconazole 2% oral gel is more useful as first-line therapy. If this fails or for children with symptoms suggestive of oesophageal candidiasis, systemic treatment with fluconazole is indicated. Resistance to the azoles can occur which will necessitate treatment with amphotericin B.

Varicella zoster virus may present with dermatomal or multidermatomal shingles or as atypical, recurrent, painful, isolated lesions. Intravenous aciclovir is required to treat younger children, but older children may respond to oral valaciclovir and this can be useful for chronic suppressive therapy. Primary infection with VZV can be complicated by respiratory failure due to pneumonitis, even with relatively high CD4 counts.

Because children very rarely complain of symptoms of unilateral eye disease, regular monitoring of severely immunocompromised children (CD4 counts $<5\%$) by an experienced ophthalmologist is desirable. Chorioretinitis due to cytomegalovirus is usually treated by intravenous induction therapy with ganciclovir followed by regular maintenance intravenous treatment five days per week. Paediatric formulations of oral ganciclovir have been poorly bioavailable to date.

Mycobacterium avium intracellulare should be considered in any child with advanced disease and a typical triad of unexplained fevers, weight loss, and abdominal discomfort. Ideally the diagnosis should be confirmed by blood culture. Life-long suppressive therapy is required using at least three drugs which should include one of the newer macrolides (clarithromycin or azithromycin) plus rifabutin plus ciprofloxacin or clofazimine or ethambutol. This may sound intolerable, but in reality such intervention can greatly improve the quality of life for the child.

Children with lymphoid interstitial pneumonitis (LIP) tend to be prone to increased chest infections, and management should be directed to prompt diagnosis and treatment of these. Inhaled steroids or bronchodilators may be useful if a reversible component is present. Treatment with systemic steroids is only indicated in the presence of hypoxia and shortness of breath, and in the absence of other respiratory pathogens. High dose oral steroids are used for up to six weeks to suppress the lymphocytic proliferation. Symptoms frequently return on weaning steroids and the lowest maintenance dose must be sought for each individual. LIP may remit spontaneously with advancing disease.

Supportive care

Unlike almost any other life-threatening disease of children, HIV simultaneously threatens the parents and other siblings. The parents' own health, their social isolation and feelings of guilt compound the difficulties of caring for a sick child. An effective well coordinated multidisciplinary team is required to address the changing needs of infected and affected children and their care givers. Continuity of care between inpatient and outpatient services, local referring hospitals, and the community needs to be developed. Ideally adults and children should be treated in family-based units. All too often parents will ignore their own health needs because they put their children first.

Confidentiality must be respected to avoid stigmatisation that may occur following disclosure of the diagnosis. The decision as to who should be informed should be tailored individually.

Families may need help in explaining the diagnosis to older children. It is not mandatory to tell staff at schools, as universal precautions should be employed for all children with cuts and abrasions. The risks of transmission from casual contacts in school or day care settings are virtually nil.

The multidisciplinary team should include a dietician, as nutritional problems and growth faltering are very common complications. Balanced supplements are frequently required and enteral feeding through gastrostomy tubes and occasionally intravenous parenteral feeding may be necessary.

The child's developmental needs require careful monitoring and support, with access to a clinical psychologist, a physiotherapist, occupational therapist and speech therapist.

Pain management is of critical importance in late stage disease. Complementary therapies such as therapeutic touch and aromatherapy may be useful and require evaluation. Skilled palliative and terminal care with flexible options for treatment at home or in the hospital or hospice are needed. Bereavement counselling for surviving family members and forward planning regarding the care of children orphaned as a result of HIV disease in parents needs to be considered. At this time, prevention is a much more realistic goal than a cure. Reducing perinatal transmission rates to below 5% is an achievable target that can only be realised if HIV-infected mothers can be identified prenatally and offered appropriate interventions. This will require a concerted effort by health professionals, public health planners, and community organisations.

13 HIV COUNSELLING AND PSYCHOSOCIAL MANAGEMENT OF AIDS PATIENTS

Lesley French, David Miller

What is Counselling?

HIV and AIDS counselling is a discussion between a client or patient and a counsellor. It may be long term or short term and has two general aims: (1) The prevention of HIV transmission, and (2) the support of those affected directly and indirectly by HIV.

Prevention counselling involves determining whether the lifestyle and behaviour of an individual or group of individuals presents them with a risk of HIV infection, working with them so that they come to understand the risks, helping to identify what meaning high-risk behaviour has for them—money, sense of group identity, and so on—helping to identify and define the true potential for behaviour change and then working to achieve and sustain appropriate and chosen changes in behaviour. This forms the basis of pretest counselling.

Supportive counselling provides help for those facing the tremendous uncertainties and stresses associated with receiving a positive result and with having HIV. Such stresses can lead to episodic or continual psychological and psychosocial morbidity in those infected and in their loved ones and carers. When counselling is not provided or is insufficient, severe, chronic psychological or psychiatric disturbance may result. Further, the patient's capacity to take up appropriate medical care may be reduced by lack of confidence in the health care system—with reduced compliance overall—where adequate preparation and support has not been given.

To avoid confusion of roles or activities, it is important to distinguish between the functions of counselling and of health education. Prevention counselling is a process of making general health education messages personally relevant so that individuals can respond in an individual way to health education that they might otherwise regard as unrealistic or of little meaning.

Counselling

- Prevention
  - determining whether the lifestyle of an individual places him or her at risk
  - working with an individual so that he or she understands the risks
  - helping to identify the meanings of high risk behaviour
  - helping to define the true potential for behaviour change
  - working with the individual to achieve and sustain appropriate and chosen behaviour
- Support
  - individual, relationship and family counselling to prevent and reduce psychological morbidity associated with HIV infection and disease

Why is counselling necessary?

It is vital that counselling should have the dual aims of prevention and support because the spread of HIV can so easily be prevented by changes in behaviour. Behaviour change can be assisted by one-to-one prevention counselling, particularly where the possibility for discussion elsewhere may be undermined by the force of social stigma. Also, when patients know that they have HIV infection or disease, they can suffer great psychosocial and psychological stresses through a fear of social stigma and rejection, a fear of disease progression and the uncertainties connected with future management of HIV. Good clinical management requires that such issues be managed with consistency and professionalism, and counselling can both minimise morbidity and reduce its likelihood.

Different HIV counselling programmes and services

- Counselling before the test is done
- Counselling after the test for those who are HIV positive and HIV negative
- Risk-reduction assessment to help and prevent transmission
- Counselling after a diagnosis of HIV disease has been made
- Family and relationship counselling
- Bereavement counselling
- Telephone "hotline" counselling
- Outreach counselling
- Crisis intervention
- Structured psychological support for those affected by HIV
- Self-help support groups

When is counselling necessary?

Pretest counselling checklist

Indications for further counselling and referral to counsellor

- Client requests to see counsellor
- Clients who appear distressed or disturbed
- Current or previous sexual partners HIV-positive
- Client presenting with clinical symptoms of HIV infection
- High-risk sexual behaviour
- High-risk injecting drug practices
- Learning or language difficulties

Points for counsellor and/or physician to cover

- What is the HIV antibody test (including seroconversion)
- The difference between HIV and AIDS
- The window period for HIV testing
- Medical advantages of knowing HIV status
- Transmission of HIV
- Safer sex and risk reduction
- Safer injecting drug use
- If the client were positive how would the client cope—support network of friends/ partner/family
- Who to tell about the test and the result
- Confidentiality of clinic records
- Insurance implications
- Does client need more time to consider
- Is further counselling indicated
- How the results of the test are obtained (in person from the physician or counsellor)

Counselling skills

- Empathy
- Non-judgemental approach
- Active listening
- Clear discussion and information giving
- Appropriate use of health education material
- Ability to develop an appropriate rapport
- Facilitating appropriate planning by enabling client decision-making
- Motivating appropriate self-care and reflection

Pretest counselling

A discussion of the implications of HIV antibody testing should accompany any offer of the test itself. This is to ensure the principle of informed consent and to assist patients to develop a realistic assessment of the risk of testing HIV antibody positive. This process should include accurate and up-to-date information about transmission and prevention of HIV and other STDs. Patients should be made aware of the "window period" for the HIV test: that a period of 12 weeks since the last possible exposure to HIV should have elapsed by the time of the test.

Patients may present for testing for any number of reasons ranging from a generalised anxiety about health to the presence of HIV-related physical symptoms. For patients at minimal risk of HIV infection, pretest counselling provides a valuable opportunity for health education and for safer sex messages to be made relevant to the individual. For patients who are at risk of HIV infection, pretest counselling is an essential part of test management. These patients may be particularly appropriate to refer for specialist counselling expertise. In genitourinary medicine clinics where HIV antibody testing is routinely offered as a part of sexual health screening, health advisers provide counselling to patients who have been identified as high risk for testing HIV positive.

The importance of undertaking a sensitive and accurate risk history of sexual partners and any injecting drug use cannot be overstated. If patients feel they cannot share this information with the physician or counsellor then the risk assessment becomes meaningless; patients may be inappropriately reassured, for example, and be unable to disclose the real reason for testing. Counselling skills are clearly an essential part of establishing an early picture of the patient and their history and of how much intervention is needed to prepare him or her for a positive result, and to further reinforce prevention messages.

Post-test counselling

Results—HIV results should be given simply, and in person. For HIV-negative patients this may be a time where the information about risk reduction can be "heard" and further reinforced. The window period of 12 weeks should be checked again and the decision taken about whether further tests for other sexually transmitted infections are appropriate.

HIV-positive patients should be allowed time to adjust to their diagnosis. Coping procedures rehearsed at the pretest counselling stage will need to be reviewed in the context of the here and now; what plans does the patient have for today, who can they be with this evening? Direct questions should be answered but the focus is on plans for the immediate few days, when further review by the counsellor should then take place. Practical arrangements including medical follow-up should be written down. Overloading the patient with information about HIV should be avoided at the result giving stage—sometimes this may happen because of the health professional's own anxiety rather than the patient's needs.

Newly diagnosed patients—Counselling support from a health adviser or specialist HIV counsellor should be available to the patient in the weeks and months following the positive test results. Immediate issues often include disclosure to others which presents complex challenges to the patient. Current and previous sexual partners at risk will have been identified at the pretest counselling stage and strategies for informing these people will be rehearsed with the counsellor. Families may be a source of support but in many instances patients need time to come to terms with their diagnosis and to fully understand its implications before they have the capacity or resources to raise it with parents, siblings, and/or loved ones who will inevitably be distressed. Being identified HIV-positive may facilitate constructive planning for the future, such as deciding on the future welfare and care of children, although this tends to happen later in the counselling process when the early shock has resolved. It is important that the perceived stigma of HIV infection is not unwittingly reinforced for newly diagnosed patients by health professionals encouraging them to be wary about telling anyone.

Counselling involves understanding a person in their social and familial contexts and many patients will derive crucial support from parents and friends. For patients who are more isolated, for whatever reason, the relationship with the counsellor can provide a high level of psychological support and strengthening of coping mechanisms during this vulnerable period. Counselling support can also help a patient engage in wider medical care and monitoring. If a person is inadequately prepared for the test, or a positive result is given inappropriately, he or she may reject further intervention and therefore the likelihood of psychological morbidity and disease progression may be increased. It seems that "getting it right" for patients at early stages of diagnosis has a profound effect upon their capacity to cope in the subsequent months and years, and to access help appropriately in later stages of disease.

Symptomatic HIV infection/diagnosis of AIDS—Most patients will remain well and asymptomatic for years after their initial infection with HIV. However, the onset of HIV-related symptoms, some of which may be classified as an AIDS diagnosis, can precipitate a psychological crisis.

Many patients who have remained well believe that illness is not going to happen to them and the resulting shock can feel as if they are being told they are HIV-positive for the first time. Many of the issues at first diagnosis will be reviewed in counselling and further decisions may be taken around disclosure to family or friends or to colleagues. The aim of counselling here is to assist the patient in adjustment and to be alert to the need for redefining support particularly in relation to community-based services such as homecare teams.

Psychological issues in HIV/AIDS counselling

(N.B. All of these may be mediated by the effects of uncertainty: see next box)

- Shock
  - of diagnosis
  - recognition of mortality
  - of loss of hope for the future
- Fear and anxiety
  - uncertain prognosis and cause of illness
  - of disfigurement and disability
  - effects of medication and treatment
  - of isolation and abandonment and social/sexual rejection
  - of infecting others and being infected by them
  - of lover's ability to cope and his or her possible illness
  - of loss of cognitive, physical, social, and work abilities
- Depression
  - over inevitability of physical decline
  - over absence of a cure
  - over the virus controlling future life
  - over limits imposed by ill health and possible social, occupational, emotional, and sexual rejection
  - from self blame and recrimination for being vulnerable to infection in the first place
- Anger and frustration
  - over inability to overcome the virus
  - over new and involuntary health/life style restrictions
- Guilt
  - interpreting HIV as a punishment; for example, for being gay or using drugs

Psychological responses

Many, indeed most, responses seen represent a normal and expected response to news of life threatening illness. More complex psychological difficulties in adjustment may indicate pre-existing morbidity and will require psychological assessment and treatment.

When a patient is found to be seropositive or diagnosed as having symptoms of HIV disease the period immediately afterwards will usually be characterised by shock, acute anxiety, depression, often impulsive despair, and social trauma. The alert physician will ensure that counselling is available at this highly vulnerable time. Patients may perceive a diagnosis of HIV infection as life threatening, and their normal psychosocial responses may, if unattended, lead to serious practical and emotional consequences, especially if the social confidentiality of the patient is not strictly preserved and continued access to counselling is denied. A complex array of emotions, including guilt about having possibly exposed partners to HIV, and anger, whether expressed or not, may predominate at this and also at later times.

People positive for HIV

Themes that arise during counselling of people positive for HIV, whether they have symptoms or not, often mimic the crisis responses to life-threatening news seen in patients with cancer but with the added pressures of social stigma and the threat of social oppression. Effective management requires allowing time for the shock of the news to sink in; there may be a period of emotional "ventilation", including overt distress. The counsellor should provide an assurance of strict confidentiality and rehearse, over time, the solutions to practical problems such as who to tell, what needs to be said, the involvement of loved ones, access to medical and dental practitioners, future sexual options, and financial and legal management. When patients are diagnosed as having HIV disease, counselling will also include discussion of possible treatment regimens and usually the question of prognosis will be raised by the patient. It is important to avoid the trap of being drawn into definitive estimates of life expectancy when there is no certainty, although patients may be well for many years. It is more appropriate to contain the immediate crisis.

With all seropositive patients it is crucial to provide a "lifeline" for the first few days (telephone numbers of the clinic, community agencies concerned with HIV, the Samaritans). Issues of disclosure need to be rehearsed at this stage in order to evaluate perceptions of likely responses to the news. Once the shock of diagnosis has abated, an appointment with a counsellor should be offered, perhaps in the company of a lover, spouse, relative or parent, within five days.

At the follow-up session issues relating to safer sex, "health boosting" (healthy eating, drinking, sleep patterns, etc.), and who should be told and how to tell them can be repeated. A partner can be involved in the counselling situation only with the consent of the patient, but it is important for the following reasons:

(1) adjustments to sexual behaviour and other lifestyle issues can be discussed and explained clearly to both;
(2) misconceptions about HIV transmission or infectiousness can be addressed;
(3) the partner's and the patient's psychological responses to the diagnoses or results, such as anxiety, depression, obsessional states, can be explained and placed in a manageable perspective.

Causes of uncertainty

- The cause of illness
  - Progression of disease
  - Forms of death and management of dying
  - Prognosis
  - Reactions of others (loved ones, employers, social networks)
- Effects of treatment
- Long-term impact of clinical trial treatments
- Disclosure impact and how this may be managed

Partners (and family members) sometimes have higher and more chronic levels of psychological morbidity arising from knowledge of HIV infection than the patients do themselves. Counselling support is often required to manage this, particularly role changes, fears about both partners being infected, and other issues may lead to difficulties in the partnership. These, in turn, may adversely affect overall management outcome.

In many cases the need for follow-up counselling may be episodic, reflecting the appearance of new or repeated infections, or the (repeated) appearance of dilemmas over involvement with clinical trials or perhaps the need for occasional reassurance over health status. The number of counselling sessions required during any of these periods largely depends on the current psychological response to infection, the physical health of the patient, the range of financial, social, domestic and other supportive resources currently available to them. At follow-up meetings it is also important to screen gently for any indications of psychological or psychiatric vulnerability. For those with HIV infection or disease there remains an often delicate dynamic tension between the processes of uncertainty and adjustment. When a lifestyle crisis emerges for those who have had HIV for many months or years, or when new diagnostic events occur, some patients may respond as they did when they were first found to have HIV.

AIDS: Safer sex guidelines for avoiding HIV

- High risk
  - unprotected anal sex
  - unprotected vaginal sex
  - sharing needles for injecting drug use
- Low risk
  - other sexual activities have minimal risk
  - there is continued debate over oral sex and HIV transmission but there is scant evidence that oral sex poses a significant risk; however, oral sex remains a source of transmission for other STDs

The worried well

Characteristics of the worried well

- Repeated negative HIV tests
- Low risk sexual history, including covert and guilt-inducing sexual activity
- Poor postadolescence sexual adjustment
- Social isolation
- Dependence in close relationships (if any)
- Multiple misinterpreted somatic features usually associated with undiagnosed viral or postviral states (not HIV) or anxiety or depression
- Psychiatric history and repeated consultation with general practitioners or physicians
- High levels of anxiety, depression and obsessional disturbance
- Increased potential for suicidal activity

Patients in this group present with multiple physical complaints which they interpret as sure evidence of their HIV infection. Typically, fears of infection reach obsessive proportions and frank obsessive and hypochondriacal states are often seen. This group shows a variety of characteristic features, and they are rarely reassured for more than a brief period after clinical or laboratory confirmation of the absence of HIV infection. In all cases a further referral for behaviourial psychotherapy or psychiatric intervention is often indicated.

Linking with community and statutory agencies

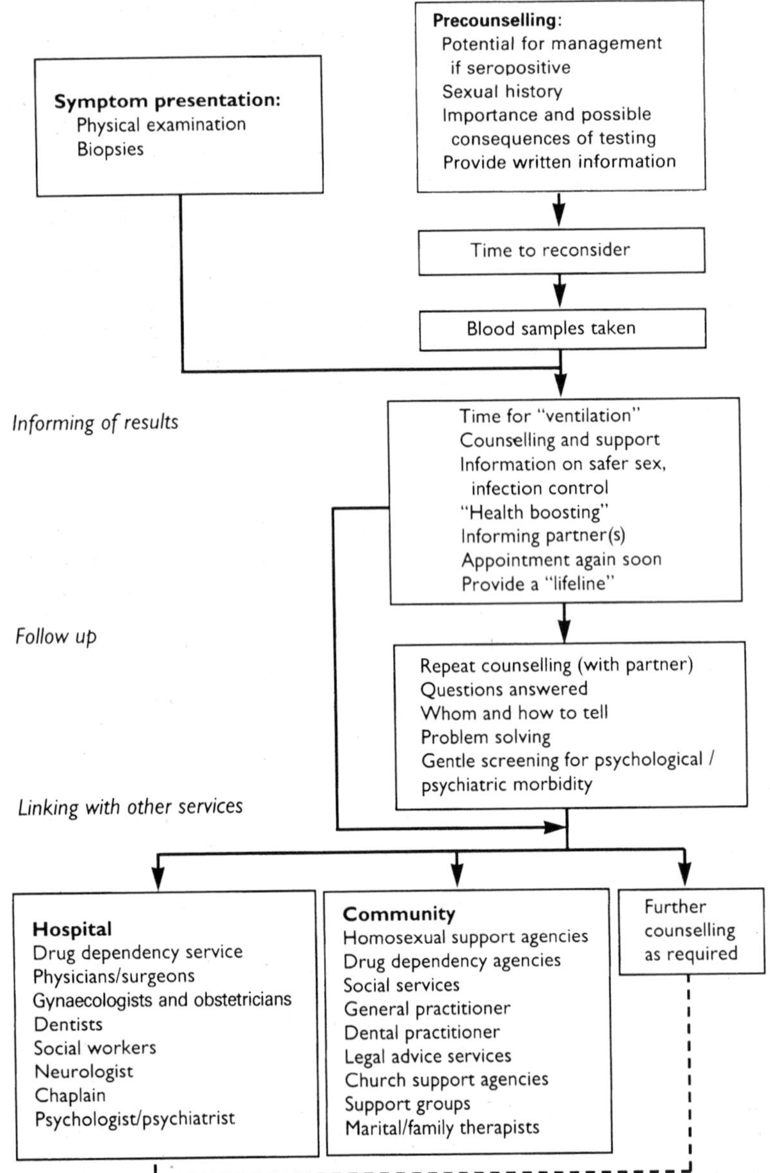

Counselling qualifications

Counselling and testing should never be provided without clear, working links with services for back-up and complementary management. Links with these services should be planned as an integral part of any HIV/AIDS counselling initiative from the outset. This is particularly important for patients from ethnic minority communities. Such links must be kept open and flexible to ensure that medical information and advice are consistent across all levels of intervention, and to enable new crises to be managed effectively as they arise. It is important, however, to ensure that roles are not unnecessarily replicated, for such replication can lead to confusion over clinical responsibilities, and worse, inconsistencies in messages given and in standards of counselling care.

Counselling in the UK is presently developing appropriate regulatory processes, but the routes to a counselling qualification remain diverse. Accordingly, the following suggestions are considered appropriate for responsible HIV counselling management:

(1) a recognised qualifying health care professional training, and formal counselling training, with an ability to use supervision appropriately;
(2) a thorough working knowledge of HIV and its clinical manifestations and an ability to keep up with developments in treatment and diagnosis in this rapidly changing area;
(3) a working knowledge of the lifestyles of patient groups and an ability to discuss sensitively issues of the patient's sexuality and lifestyle;

Who is HIV and AIDS counselling for?

- People worried that they might have HIV
- People considering being tested for HIV
- People who have been tested for HIV (infected and non-infected)
- People choosing not to be tested despite past or present risk behaviour
- People unaware of the risks involved in behaviours that they are, or have been, engaged in
- People with HIV infection and disease, including AIDS
- People experiencing practical and emotional difficulties as a result of HIV infection
- Family, loved ones, friends and colleagues of people with HIV
- Health workers and others in regular contact with people with HIV

(4) a working knowledge of the range of "back-up" services available for patients with HIV infection and AIDS together with the ability to communicate effectively, tactfully, and sympathetically with people from a wide variety of backgrounds and lifestyles;
(5) the ability to recognise common psychosocial and clinical complications arising from HIV infection, including anxiety, depression, obsessive disorders, neurological indications, and suicidal risk.

If counsellors cannot manage such issues themselves, they must be able to recognise when to refer patients elsewhere.

Forms of psychosocial and stress management

Coping strategies

- Using counselling
- Problem solving
- Participation in discussions about treatment
- Recreation and socialising
- Use of alternative therapies, for example relaxation massage
- Exploring potential for control over manageable issues
- Disclosure of HIV status and using support options

The importance of encouraging and working towards coping strategies involving active participation (to the extent the patient can manage) in planning of care and in seeking appropriate social support has been demonstrated clinically and empirically. Such an approach includes encouraging problem-solving, participation in treatment, decision making, active distractions through recreation and socialising, and emphasising self-worth and the potential for personal control over manageable issues in life. Finally, the value of groups in HIV psychosocial and stress management is amply demonstrated. Groups are valuable in reducing an individual's sense of isolation—of being the only one—in providing a safe place to express feelings, to share experiences, and to learn successful coping styles from others. They, therefore, have a very constructive social support function and may help in risk reduction by establishing and emphasising an ethos of safer sex or safer injecting drug use. They also provide a forum for stress management to be demonstrated, along with the skills necessary for accessing appropriate social and practical supports. To date, reports have emphasised the value of groups in stress management with gay men, with sharing coping experiences with people with HIV, and with managing AIDS-related bereavement.

Future directions in HIV counselling

Counselling in HIV and AIDS has become a foundation element in a model of care in which psychological issues are recognised as integral to patient management. In the absence of empirical data, counselling has remained a core clinical activity in HIV management, largely because patients continue to request and assert its value. However, the need for quantitative data on the value of HIV counselling is pressing. Outcome studies emphasising patient-identified indicators in measuring efficacy, alongside "conventional" outcomes, will be required if conclusions are to reflect adequately the true value and meaning of counselling for patients.

The need to provide opportunities for counselling for HIV staff is increasingly being recognised as a useful element of standard occupational care. As the stresses of HIV work are becoming better characterised, particularly in areas of high HIV prevalence, the need to employ systems to retain experienced staff who may otherwise be lost through occupational morbidity is increasingly important, as are programmes of staff support and stress management.

Finally, significant developments in anti-retroviral therapy have led to a surge of optimism about long term medical management of HIV infection. However, efficacy of drug regimens depend on patient compliance, where drugs have to be taken several times a day, some with food, others on an empty stomach and so on. Much uncertainty remains about long term efficacy. Counselling may be an important tool in determining a realistic assessment of individual compliance and in supporting the complex adjustment to a daily routine of medication.

14 PALLIATIVE CARE AND PAIN CONTROL

Rob George, Nina Swire

Someone once said "If we can get it right for AIDS, we can get it right for everything". In effectively caring for those patients in whom death is almost certain and not too far off we have to face the challenge of integrating the grey area between acute and palliative practice. Assessment and control of physical, psychological or emotional, and spiritual distress becomes as much a priority as good medical management. This ideal is complicated by the coping strategies of denial, among both patients and family, and practitioners. This propagates the many misconceptions in palliative care. In short *palliative* (symptom-based) and *therapeutic* (pathology-based) approaches are not mutually exclusive. Patients facing chronic ill health, or those with acute, highly symptomatic disease may benefit from specialist advice or shared care as much as those in the terminal phase of their illness.

Myths to be broken

- Fighters want treatment, failures want palliation
- "Tablets of stone" philosophy; once decided, strategies cannot be changed
- "There is nothing more that we can do"

The therapeutic dilemma

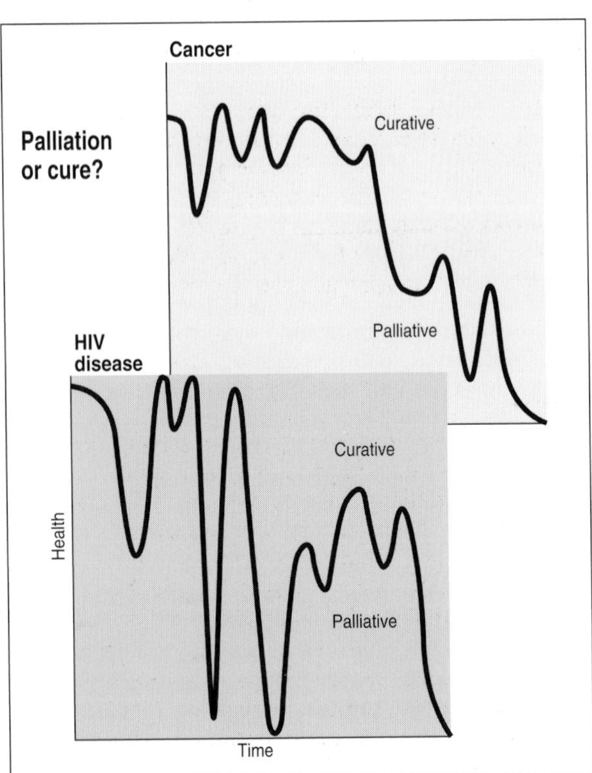

Differences between palliation and cure in HIV and cancer.

In the case of HIV disease, even after AIDS has been diagnosed, t biggest problem is the unpredictability of disease progression. Wher this syndrome is universally fatal with life-threatening opportunistic infections, malignancies, and frequent progressive neurological diseas or wasting, in most cases intercurrent illnesses are interspersed with background of relatively stable health. Although each supervening illness generally weakens and debilitates the patient, recovery may le to months of good quality living. In this respect, it is different to cancer, where the progression of disease is more predictable and the respective place of curative and palliative care is clearer.

Thus the distinction between palliation and cure is often blurred. Active treatment regularly continues alongside palliative measures: firstly with aggressive and potentially curative therapy during acute episodes, and secondly with prophylactic and maintenance regimens try and maintain residual health. However, in the light of approachi death it is important to consider not only the clinical needs of the patient but also the potential costs and benefits of any intervention i personal terms.

The quantity/quality equation

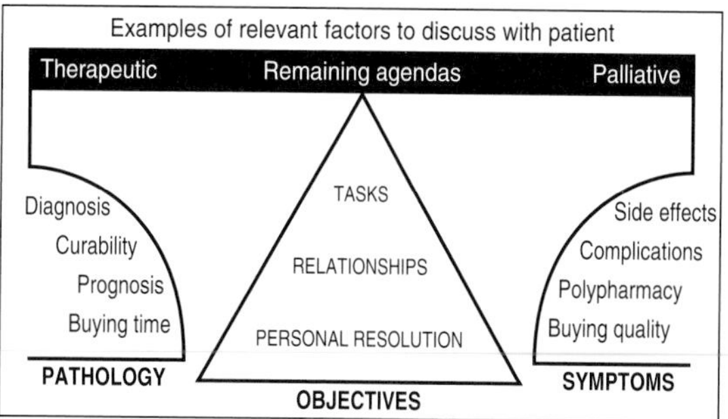

Treatment: applying a cost-benefit ratio.

The dying patient's priorities may be very different from the clinician's. As disease advances, and quality of life generally becomes more important than its quantity, the need to balance these costs and benefits increases: in particular, the patient's willingness to accept the side effects of an intervention, whether diagnostic or therapeutic. Certainties such as time and energy expended on a course of treatment or immediate and short-term benefits, become increasingly important in decision-making.

Try not to make assumptions about a patient's views or wishes. The subtle ways in which illness and the individual interact mean that social, psychological, and spiritual elements may be every bit as relevant as the underlying pathology. Discuss the issues with the patient individually, trusting that those not wanting to be involved in decision-making will let you know.

Working with the dying

The patient is at the centre of decision-making

- Work in partnership with the patient and family
- Share responsibility for making decisons
- Maximise the patient's control over decision-making
- Work in a positive framework
- Agree specific tasks
- Set realistic goals
- Review regularly
- Remain open to creative options

Partnership

Practically, set goals and objectives with the patient and operate within that framework. Strategies should be examined regularly. Aggressive treatment to reach a specific goal should be reviewed immediately that objective is met—a patient's wishes may have been altered radically as a result of success or failure. Be realistic, yet at the same time be prepared to allow a patient to risk things such as travel provided they are well informed. Above all plan positively: people wish to live until they die. One of the greatest fears for the dying is helplessness. The more a patient and family feel their agendas, wishes, and hopes are being taken seriously, the better they are able to cope.

Answering questions about prognosis

- Choose a "safe" place
- Include significant others and/or other professionals
- Explore the patient's understanding
- Be honest: don't collude with unrealistic hopes and don't be afraid to say "I don't know"
- Be kind: allow the patient to set the limits on the discussion when exploring painful truths
- Arrange a future contact

Discussing prognosis

Open sharing of information inevitably leads to questions about prognosis. Always speak to individuals where they are able to express emotions openly. Never do this in an open ward. Include significant others if possible and invite another professional (for example the key nurse), who can reinforce the discussion and offer support.

In order to gauge the level of knowledge, anxiety, or fear that the person has, explore their understanding of the situation carefully in the light of previous information. Start the conversation in an open way; for example "As I am sure you know, this illness is very unpredictable and I think the situation has changed quite a lot since you last had a conversation like this."

According to the stage of illness, break the future into tangible and appropriately small blocks of time such as one to three months. The intervals chosen will depend on each case. Confine your prognostication to this period and use general terms such as better, the same or worse. Always say that the unexpected may happen. If possible, arrange to review the discussion over the following few days in order to answer outstanding questions. This will also provide the opportunity to revise an opinion.

Symptom control

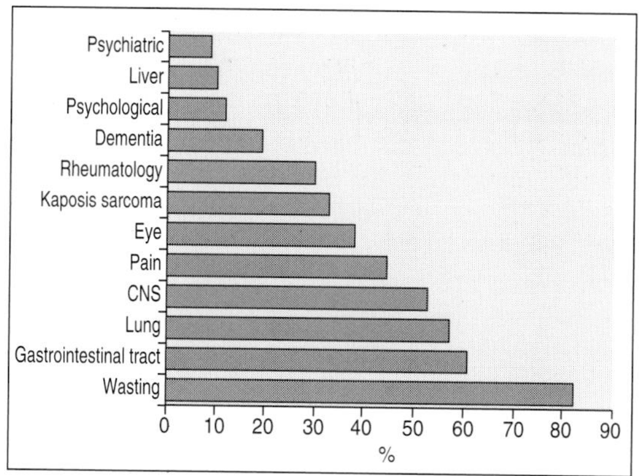

Symptoms and systems involved in last three months.

The significance of symptoms

Many patients are fearful of pain and loss of dignity during the dying process. They and their families can gain much psychological benefit knowing that expert help is available to treat or palliate their physical symptoms effectively and to help them address psychological, social and existential/spiritual issues. In regard to symptom control one of the most important concepts we can put across is the hope that there is always something more we can do, *not* that the disease and death will go away.

Intervention may be unconventional, for example using a drug for its side effect rather than its accustomed indication. Opiates are the classic example: traditionally used as analgesics, their central effects on breathing pattern and respiratory drive and their peripheral action as constipating agents are of great benefit in reducing dyspnoea and controlling diarrhoea.

Fundamentals of pain management

- Any pain, however generated, is a genuine symptom
- Always assume that there is a physical trigger, until proven otherwise
- The vast majority of patients have a combination of pain types

Incidence

A wide spectrum of symptoms occur in HIV disease and many patients will have multiple symptomatology (75% of patients have two or more symptoms). Pain problems are common, affecting at least 60% in the terminal stages. Noxious and debilitating symptoms, especially pain, adversely impact on quality of life and are significant risk factors for depression and suicide. They need to be treated aggressively.

Pain management is the most important palliative skill and will be dealt with in some detail. However, the choices, combinations, and doses of drugs are empirical, but palliation is not limited to this symptom. Further information can be found in other texts listed at the end of this chapter.

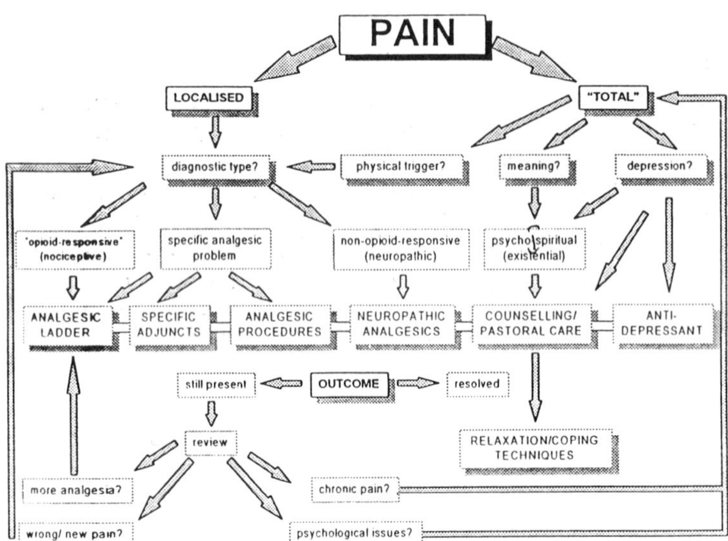

Therapeutic approach to pain.

Pain control

Effective pain management requires diagnosis, as neuropathic and emotional pain in particular need specific approaches. Traditionally, pain is categorised according to its response to opioids.

Oral morphine facts

- Dose range is 1000-fold: (2·5 mg every 4 hours to 2·5 g every 4 hours or more)
- The majority of patients require $<$200 mg/day
- It is not addictive when used therapeutically

Opioid responsive pain—Opioid responsive pain is caused by local tissue damage (nociceptive, somatic, and viscera pain). It responds to non-steroidal anti-inflammatory drugs (NSAIDs), opiates, fentanyl, and the newer analgesics such as ketoralac (an anti-inflammatory with potent, non-opioid analgesic properties); 90% of such pains are controllable using the analgesic ladder.

The analgesic ladder

- Bottom rung
  - non-narcotic: aspirin, paracetamol, NSAIDs

  Don't underestimate these drugs, they are important in their own right
- Middle rung
  - weak narcotic: codeine, dextropropoxyphene, oxycodone
- Upper rung
  - strong narcotic: morphine, papaveretum, phenazocine, etc.

  ⇒ *Use adjuvant medication in combination*
  ⇒ *If a drug fails to relieve, do not move laterally, move up the ladder*

GI prophylaxis with NSAIDs

- H_2-receptor antagonist
- Proton pump inhibitor
- Prostaglandin analogue, either as single agent or as compound preparation such as Arthrotec (Diclofenac/misoprostol)

The analgesic ladder

Bottom rung—Paracetamol and NSAIDs may provide adjuvant analgesia even in patients needing strong opiates. Remember, paracetamol influences other drugs' metabolism, specifically, in HIV disease, that of zidovudine. However, in general, palliative physicians would be happy to use doses up to 6 g/day (the BNF recommends 4 g/24 hours). Similarly, gastrointestinal complications (use appropriate prophylaxis) or renal impairment with NSAIDs should not be absolute contraindications in patients with short prognosis and severe pain.

Middle rung—The weak opiates, codeine-based drugs or compound analgesics (co-codamol, co-dydramol etc.), may be helpful for mild to moderate pain. Formulations differ slightly in efficacy and prescribing is essentally empirical. Alternatively, a small dose of a strong opioid can be used. Whilst tolerance and dependence are well documented in a minority, taking opioids chronically causes addiction in $\leqslant$0·1%.

Upper rung—Many strong opiates are available, various analogues expressing side effects and analgesia (potency and half-life) in differing degrees. Morphine is the drug of choice by mouth. Use alternative opioids or fentanyl *only* where there is a specific problem with morphine. Alternatively side effects may be reduced by using co-analgesics.

Opioid side effects

- Nausea and vomiting: dose-related
  - chemorecepter trigger zone and vestibular stimulation

  ⇒ *Prescribe anti-emetics routinely for the first five days*

- Constipation: may be desirable, dose-related
  - peripheral effect

  ⇒ *Always prescribe laxatives*

- Clouding of consciousness: hallucinations rare
  - central effect, fades with time

  ⇒ *Always warn the patient of initial drowsiness*

- Respiratory depression: good for dyspnoea
  - central + peripheral cough suppression pain has a partially protective effect

  ⇒ *Increase dose carefully where chronic lung disease present*

Dealing with opiate toxicity

- The half life of morphine and diamorphine is four hours
- Respiratory rates down to 5 or 10 are acceptable for a few hours
- Central effects can be antagonised, but will lead to rebound agitation and hyperresponsiveness

  ⇒ *It is best simply to stop the opiate and wait*

In extremis

⇒ *Naloxone* is the specific antidote and reverses all the actions of opiates; use very small doses
⇒ *Physostigmine* can be used to selectively antagonise respiratory depression
⇒ *Amphetamines* can successfully counteract drowsiness

Opiate toxicity

Patient response to opioids is idiosyncratic. For some the therapeutic window may be very small. In poorly controlled pain (usually non-opioid responsive), escalating doses may lead to opiate toxicity: confusion, hallucinations, agitation, and myoclonic jerks. Paradoxical pain (loss of analgesia and increasing pain) may occur. If not corrected, unconsciousness and death from respiratory depression ensues. Confusion in the dying is complex and increasing opiates is not the only solution to increasing pain. You may need to stop all opiates until symptoms have subsided. *Seek the advice of an expert.*

Good prescribing

Good prescribing in pain control

- Always prescribe regular analgesia, at intervals appropriate to drug pharmacokinetics
- "p.r.n." Analgesia is for breakthrough pain only

Neuropathic pain

- Generated in nervous system
- Source can be local nerve to thalamus
- Caused by:
  - toxins (chemotherapy)
  - invasion/compression (tumour)
  - damage by viruses (HSV, CMV, HIV)
  - demyelination of any kind
- Often coexists with nociceptive pain
- May not present with classical dysaesthesia
- Seldom opioid responsive

Opioid responsive pain can normally be controlled within 24 to 48 hours. Morpine should be titrated using immediate release formulations (for example, Oramorph elixir, Sevredol tablets). Their effect peaks within the hour and last four hours. Titrate with a four-hourly regime with "top-ups" for breakthrough pain: 25–50% of dose and a 25–50% increase in the next scheduled dose as necessary. In individuals with hepatic or renal impairment, the increases should proceed more slowly. Slow-release preparations (for example, MST b.d. or MXL o.d.) are best for maintenance. The immediate release formulations should continue to be available for breakthrough pain at a dose at least one sixth of the final 24-hour dose.

Opioid non-responsive pain—Neuropathy is the most important cause of partial or absent opioid responsiveness. It is a common complication of HIV and may be very difficult to relieve. Any opioid response usually needs doses disproportionate to the pain.

Neuropathic analgesics

- Tricyclic antidepressants:
  - lofepramine (70 mg 1–3 times/day)
  - amitriptyline (10–150 mg nocte +/− day time doses)
- Anticonvulsants:
  - carbamazepine (start dose of 100 mg b.d. up to 1600 mg day)
  - valproate (200–1200 mg/day)
  - phenytoin (up to 300 mg per day)
- Benzodiazepines:
  - clonazepam (0·5–4 mg nocte)
  - diazepam, midazolam (parenterally)
- Membrane stabilisers:
  - flecainide (100–200 mg b.d.)
  - lignocaine (s.c. or i.v. infusion in doses of 0·5 mg/kg/h)
- Others:
  - clonidine, octreotide; seek advice

Drugs affecting nerve conduction or nerve-blocking techniques usually work. However, choices, combinations, and doses, are empirical, especially as individual response appears to be arbitrary even within groups: for example, a patient may gain no benefit from amitriptyline but be significantly helped with lofepramine. Secondly, benefit may take several days to gain. Thirdly, neuropathic analgesics have significant and potentially dose-limiting side effects and dose increases should be made slowly. Patient, family, and staff may need support in keeping a steady hand whilst the best combinations are found.

Intractable cases or root or cord problems may need a nerve block or long-term epidural. Many different techniques are available. They carry potential morbidity, so use cost:benefit analysis with the patient to decide a plan. *Don't make choices on behalf of the patient; immobility and incontinence free of pain may be a valid choice.*

Oesophageal and rectal pain and spasm

- Treat primary pathology (including constipation)
- Smooth muscle relaxant
  - nifedipine (5–20 mg); fast. If effective use regularly
- Anticholinergics
  - hyoscine as Kwells sublingually, patch or injection (also antiemetic)
- Irritation
  - H_2 receptor antagonist, proton pump inhibitor or carbenoxolone prophylaxis in oesophageal disease
  - in rectal/anal disease prescribe lignocaine gel p.r.n.

Opioid partially-responsive pains

This comprises those pains that fluctuate and are difficult to control with long-acting maintenance regimens, or have components which are non-opioid responsive, Their treatment requires accurate diagnosis and the use of specific "adjuvants". Morphine may play a part in their management.

The gut—

- Oesophageal pain can be very severe and frequently includes spasm indistinguishable from cardiac pain.
- Reflux often worsens the situation.
- Any rectal pathology can cause tenesmus.
- Colic and visceral pains are almost always opioid responsive but may need specific anticholinergic adjuncts, such as hyoscine or buscopan.

Wound pain—This is of relevance in problems such as ulcerating Kaposi's sarcoma. These pains may combine nociception and neuropathy as well as episodes of acute exacerbation. Background analgesia, topical and episodic "top-up" may all be needed.

Wound pain

- Treat infection
  - metronidazole gel topically
  - systemic antibiotics
- Systemic analgesia
  - morphine regularly
  - dextromoramide (Palfium) for procedures
- Topical anaesthetics
  - marcaine 0·25–0·75% soaked dressings; need daily dressings to maintain benefit
- Benzydamine (NSAID/local anaesthetic)
  - 3% aqueous cream absorbed transdermally

SYMPTOMS
DISFIGUREMENT
SIDE-EFFECTS
Absent friends
Absent family
Tired of life
Future
Incurability
PROGNOSIS
LOSS
THE DISEASE
Professional incompetence
No more treatment
Income
Sleeplessness
Irritability
DEPRESSION
ANGER
TOTAL PAIN
Role
Wasted time
ANTICIPATORY GRIEF
INSUFFICIENT TIME
Guilt
Prestige
LOSS OF CONTROL
Unforgiveness
Worth
ANXIETY
FEARS
Future
Sense of self
Financial pressure
Dependency
Denial
Family burden
UNCERTAINTY
HELPLESSNESS
DEATH
Pain
God?
Loneliness
"being sent away"
Dying process
Conflict
Rejection

Total body pain.

Total body pain

This is the difficult area of suffering and the subtle interactions of our psyche, beliefs, and body. Some people use the terms "soul", "emotional", or "spiritual" pain. Suffering can be vented physically through other symptoms such as nausea or bowel disturbance, but pain is by far the commonest vehicle of somatisation. It is complex, distressing, and very real. It stems from a lowered threshold of distress to the given symptom or pathology. For understandable reasons, there is always an element of this in any dying person as they process and face their death and what it means. Fear and guilt are the common roots for many. Don't forget, *paene* (punishment) is the latin root of pain.

Effective management requires one to deal, not only with any physical component but, also with the meaning of the symptomatology and the exacerbating effects of fear, anxiety, sleeplessness, loss of future, and of death and its connotations for the individual. In this difficult area do not be afraid to refer for help from a counsellor, psychologist, or spiritual adviser.

As death approaches

Preterminal restlessness

- Exclude urinary retention
- Treat any suspected pain
- Check that there is not an important visitor that the patient must see or hear
- Check for an important date or anniversary
- Exclude any important religious rite
- Sedate as necessary: midazolam (starting at 10–100 mg/24 hours), methotrimeprazine (12·5–300 mg/24 hours)

General points

If anything, this is the most critical time of management for staff, patient, and relatives. It is a source of enduring memory. The last few days well managed often compensate for times of distress and disorder in the final months of a person's life. They leave everyone with a sense of completion and accurate feeling that a patient's struggle in the face of deteriorating health to "make sense" and "stave off the inevitable" have come together and been "worthwhile".

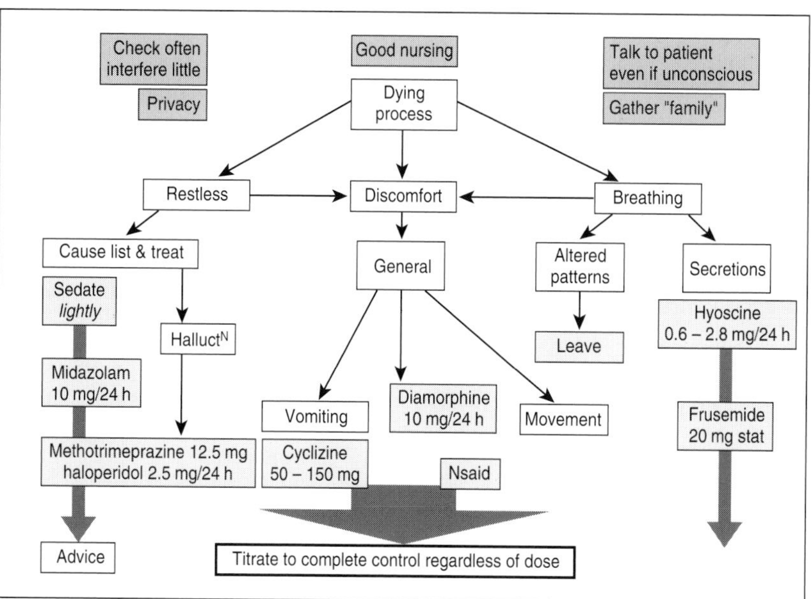

Patient management in final few days.

Being the "true physician"

Pragmatism and sensitivity are of increasing importance. Patients experience increasing loss of appetite, weakness, and somnolence (and in the terminal phase unconsciousness and altered breathing patterns). Be calm and reassuring: explain that these changes are normal, to be expected and don't cause physical suffering, because they don't. Time and patience with the family and one's nursing colleagues is invaluable to them and relieve anxiety. It is a time to be a fellow human being, recognise that we will all face this ourselves and there is no shame in witnessing, sharing, or expressing the feeling that accompany the hours of a person's parting.

Being the practical physician

Most importantly continue to visit. The clinical situation can change very quickly. Assess symptoms regularly and change palliative therapeutics as necessary (even several times a day). As swallowing becomes difficult swap to *par rectum* or *parenteral* routes. With the limited communication, problems may manifest themselves as *preterminal restlessness* or distress. Possible physical and psychological/spiritual triggers need to be checked and acted on.

In general, encourage the family to talk normally to the patient and to say whatever they need to say. Reassure them that the patient can hear and continue to explain all that you do to the patient and chat normally through procedures. Your patient is not dead yet, and may actually be very aware, so treat him with the dignity that he deserves.

This period of life, when the dying process is actively underway, may be short-lived or take many days. In most cases whatever is taking place is not known to us. Where beliefs are unknown or unfamiliar it is best presented neutrally as a time of transition; our place is to care.

A simple approach to the last few days is given in the final figure.

Conclusions

Managing the young dying is difficult, of that there is no doubt. However, if one understands and accepts that there comes a time when technology and acute strategies take second place to good symptom control and general, sensitive medicine, then one's practice gains a depth and relevance that can only enrich oneself, one's patients and restore the art of our profession.

15 CONTROL OF INFECTION POLICIES

D J Jeffries, C A Aitken

Intensive epidemiological studies of HIV infection have shown that it is not transmitted in the community by casual or intimate non-sexual contact.

As of December 1995 there have been 79 documented instances of confirmed occupational transmission of HIV of which 76 were in health care workers and three were in non-clinical laboratory workers. There have been, in addition, 144 cases of HIV infection, possibly resulting from occupational transmission in exposed individuals with no other known risk of infection. The rate of transmission after a single percutaneous exposure to HIV positive material is 0·32% (21 confirmed infections after 6 498 exposures in 25 studies). The risk of infection after exposure of mucous membranes and/or conjunctivae to infected material is 0·03% (one confirmed infection after 2 885 exposures in 21 studies).

It is important to design infection control policies which, while protecting staff against the risk of infection, do not compromise medical and dental care. HIV is one of several blood-borne viruses; carriers of these viruses may be perfectly well and individuals may be unaware that they are infected. Some, including the hepatitis viruses B and C are potentially more infectious than HIV. Thus, health care workers and society in general need to adjust to the concept that direct contact with the blood of others may present a potential, albeit low, risk of infection.

In the UK the Department of Health and many other bodies have issued guidelines to educate and protect health care and community workers. Awareness of the risks, education, careful attention to work practices, provision of protective equipment, and immunisation against hepatitis B, where appropriate, are measures which will reduce to a minimum the risk of infection with all blood-borne viruses.

Selected guidelines

- United Kingdom Health Departments. *Guidance for clinical health care workers: protection against infection with HIV and hepatitis viruses. Recommendations of the Expert Advisory Group on AIDS.* London: HMSO, January 1990.
- *A Code of Practice for sterilisation of instruments and control of cross infection.* London: British Medical Association, June 1989.
- *The safe disposal of clinical waste.* London: HMSO, 1982.
- United Kingdom Health Departments—AIDS/HIV Infected Health Care Workers. *Guidance on the management of infected health care workers. Recommendations of the Expert Advisory Group on AIDS.* London: DOH, March 1994.
- Advisory Committee on Dangerous Pathogens. *Protection against bloodborne infections in the workplace: HIV and hepatitis.* London, HMSO, 1995.
- Royal College of Pathologists. *HIV and the practice of pathology.* London: Marks & Spencer Publication Unit of the Royal College of Pathologists, July 1995.

Hospital care

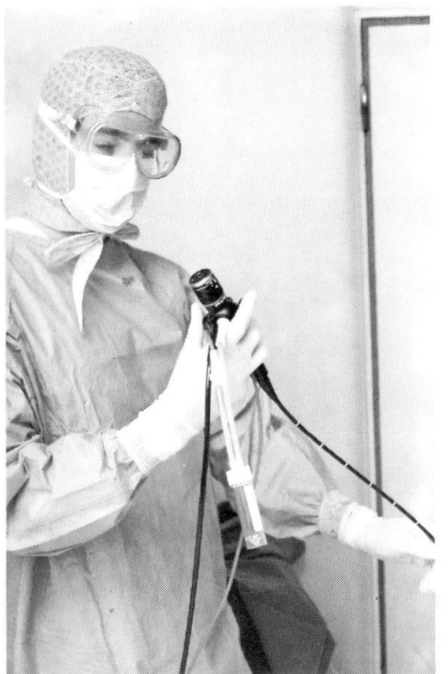

Bronchoscopy in a patient infected with HIV.

HIV positivity *per se* is not an indication for isolating a patient. It may be necessary to consider source isolation, however, if there is evidence of active infection with other agents, such as *Mycobacterium tuberculosis*, varicella-zoster virus, or salmonella, or if there is a likelihood of extensive exposure to body fluids from, for example, haemorrhage or severe diarrhoea.

Medical practices should be of a sufficiently high standard to eliminate any risk of patient-to-patient spread of HIV in hospital. This is achieved, as part of general infection control procedures, by using disposables, and by paying careful attention to decontamination and sterilisation. Attempts to recycle disposables or to bypass accepted disinfection procedures may lead to nosocomial infection.

Staff should adopt sensible precautions if contamination with blood or other body fluids is likely. This applies particularly for the management of known virus carriers but should also be the routine for any patient. The concept of "universal precautions" for all patients is being introduced increasingly into health care. In most cases precautions entail no more than wearing disposable gloves and an apron, but in certain circumstances, such as bronchoscopy, protective spectacles and a mask may be necessary to protect the eyes and mouth. Most aspects of patient care and examination do not expose the staff to body fluids, and protective clothing is not required.

Many staff sustain inoculation injuries while manipulating needles and sharp instruments. Education and careful attention to technique will reduce the risks to a minimum. No attempt should be made to resheathe needles unless a safe resheathing device is available, and needles should be placed immediately into safe sharps disposal containers.

Although there is little epidemiological evidence of increased risk, many hospitals assume that special care should be taken during surgery on known or suspected HIV carriers. This usually means adopting pre-existing policies for hepatitis B carriers and may include the introduction of double-gloving and additional protective clothing. Preventing unnecessary exposure to body fluids and trying to reduce the incidence of penetrating injuries to a minimum are the best defence against infections, which may be present, but unsuspected, in any patient.

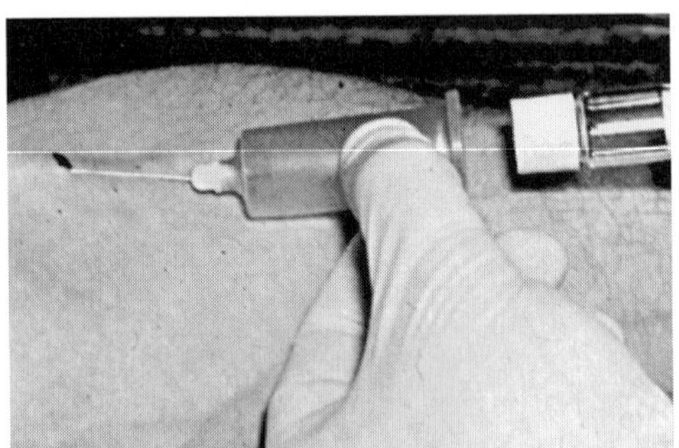

A vacuum collection system of the type shown reduces the risk of spillage when large volumes of blood are required.

Reports of transmission of HIV from a dentist to his patients have raised public concerns about the risks of acquiring HIV and other blood-borne viruses from health care workers. Guidelines produced by th UK Health Departments identify work practices known as "exposure-prone invasive procedures" as aspects of medical care that present a potential risk of transfer of a blood-borne virus from health care workers to patients.

Exposure-prone procedures are those where there is a risk that injury to the worker may result in the exposure of the patient's open tissue to the blood of the worker. These procedures include those where the worker's gloved hands may be in contact with sharp instruments, needle tips, or sharp tissues (spicules of bone or teeth) inside a patient's open body cavity, wound, or confined anatomical space where the hands or fingertips may not be completely visible at all times.

Health care workers who are either HIV positive or "infectious" carriers of hepatitis B virus (HBeAg positive) are excluded from exposure-prone procedures. Follow-up studies of patients who have undergone surgery by HIV positive surgeons have all been negative, although there are many reports of hepatitis B transmission from staff to patients. Clearly, the risks to the patient from HIV in health care workers are extremely low but the frequency of inoculation injury to the surgeon during the course of major surgery highlights the need for continued surveillance.

Sharps disposal

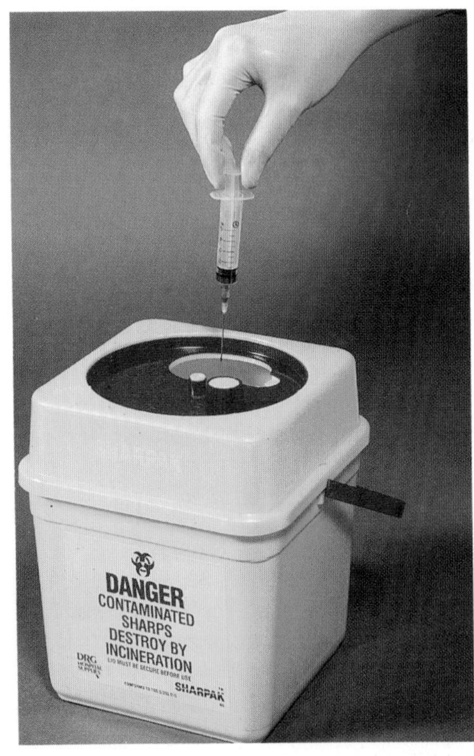

Safe sharps disposal.

Clinical laboratory staff are at risk from certain pathogens which may be present in specimens. The Advisory Committee on Dangerous Pathogens originally produced specific guidelines for work on samples from HIV positive patients. These have now been reissued to encompass potential risks from all blood-borne viruses. The most important aspects of safety in the laboratory are education, training, and prevention of inoculation and skin contact with body fluids. It is important to review all laboratory procedures to reduce the use of needles and the danger of exposure to glass fragments. This may necessitate increased investment in automatic pipetting systems to replace the need for glass pipettes. The absence of evidence of airborne transmission means that HIV positive samples may be handled on the open bench providing the work is conducted in optimal facilities and the operator is free from distraction and disturbance. The current practice of alerting laboratory staff to samples from known or suspected HIV positive patients by the use of biohazard stickers may be defended on the basis that it reduces risks. It must, however, be emphasised constantly that in the present epidemic no unfixed specimens can be considered free from infection.

Community aspects

Community aspects of decontamination

- Cutlery, crockery, clothing
  - decontaminated by normal washing
- Decontaminate blood spillages with bleach (hypochlorite)

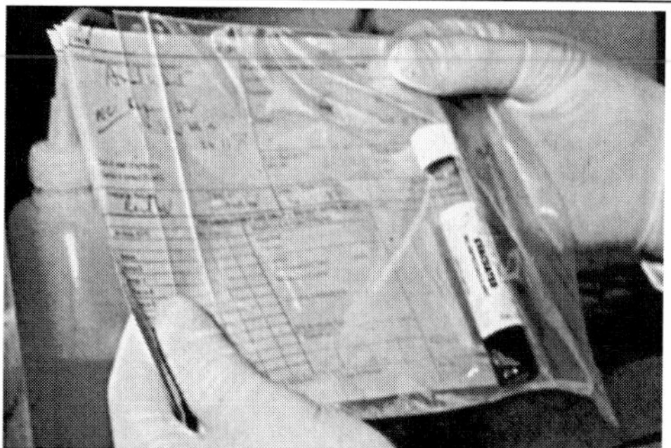

Secure bagging for specimen and request sent to laboratory.

HIV carriers in the community present no risk to others from normal day-to-day contact. The combined effects of dilution, temperature, and detergent action ensure that standard washing procedures will satisfactorily decontaminate cutlery, crockery, and clothing. All blood spillages should be decontaminated with hypochlorite (bleach) and carefully cleaned up. The absence of evidence that saliva can transmit HIV means that nobody should withhold mouth-to-mouth resuscitation from someone who has suffered a respiratory arrest. Members of the rescue services who frequently carry out resuscitation, often in cases in which facial injury exposes them to blood as well as saliva, are provided with devices. Anyone attempting to use a resuscitation device must be adequately trained as, in the wrong hands, it may prejudice the life of the casualty and in some cases increase the potential risks to the operator by causing bleeding.

Disinfection

An important method of reducing the potential infectivity of viruses is dilution. Thus procedures such as thorough cleaning and handwashing are central to any infection control policy and must never be neglected. HIV has been described as a fragile virus, and this is true to an extent. Although it is effectively inactivated by many different agents, survival of virus may be prolonged at ambient temperatures, and infectious virus may still be present in dried blood after a week. This means that any surfaces and fomites that have been in contact with clinical material must be decontaminated.

The trend towards the use of disposables reduces the need for decontamination in many areas. Thorough cleaning followed by heat sterilisation should be adopted, if at all possible, for any reusable equipment. Although HIV is inactivated by boiling, autoclaving has become the norm in clinical practice. With increasing numbers of HIV carriers in the community it is important for their protection to ensure that instruments are rendered free of all organisms, including bacterial and fungal spores. Organisms that may present no risk to people with normal immunity may lead to opportunistic infections if they are immunocompromised by HIV infection or other agents such as chemotherapeutic drugs.

Disinfection

- Autoclave or use disposables if possible
- Hypochlorite (1000 ppm available chlorine) for general decontamination
- Hypochlorite (10 000 ppm available chlorine) if organic matter, including blood, present
- 2% Glutaraldehyde (freshly activated) N.B. Beware of dangerous fumes.

Liquid disinfectants must always be considered a poor alternative to heat sterilisation. Difficulties exist in controlling their potency, most are caustic, and most are rapidly inactivated by organic matter. For hospital or community use, if it is necessary to use a liquid disinfectant, it is sensible to choose one which is known to inactivate hepatitis B and other pathogens such as *Mycobacterium tuberculosis*, as well as HIV.

All waste that is contaminated with blood must be considered potentially infective and treated as "clinical waste" in accordance with the Health Services Advisory Committee's document *The safe disposal of clinical waste*. Sharps containers must meet Department of Health specifications and must be incinerated before disposal.

First aid and inoculation injuries

First aid

- Body fluids on skin, in eyes, or in mouth
  - wash away immediately
- Penetrating wounds
  - encourage bleeding
  - wash with soap and water
  - report to supervisor and medical officer

In the event of exposure to blood, simple first-aid measures should be applied immediately. Any blood or other body fluids on the skin should be washed away with soap and water. Splashes into the mouth or eye should be diluted by washing, and sterile eye-wash bottles should be provided in any areas where this is likely to occur. A skin puncture should be encouraged to bleed in an attempt to express any material deposited in the wound. The wound should then be washed thoroughly. Any injury to a member of staff should be reported immediately to the person in charge and then to the occupational health physician or other medical adviser. In hospital this allows for the opportunity to investigate the state of health of the person inoculated and, if necessary, to take protective measures such as hepatitis B prophylaxis or antibiotic cover, or the use of antiretroviral drugs such as zidovudine. The medical adviser should discuss whether blood samples should be taken for future reference of HIV testing and whether a programme of follow-up consultations should be started.

Those concerned with counselling people who have sustained inoculation injuries should have enough knowledge to provide current information about the risks of occupational exposure and should be able to advise on changes in lifestyle such as the adoption of safer sex practices.

In summary, the risk of transmission of HIV within hospitals and to carers in the community is low. Education of staff, good infection control procedures, and safe working practices can help to minimise this risk. Due attention to these measures at all times will ensure the protection of patients and staff.

16 STRATEGIES FOR PREVENTION

Anne M Johnson, Michael W Adler

General health education

Health promotion activity

- General health education
- Information, counselling, and HIV antibody testing
- Screening of blood and organ donations
- Heat treatment of blood products
- Protection of health care staff
- Surveillance

Health promotion activity aimed at changing behaviour remains the major preventive strategy for reducing the spread of HIV. Although research continues, there is no immediate prospect for cure or vaccine.

The pioneers of health promotion campaigns in the United States and Britain have been voluntary groups, initially directing their efforts towards homosexual men. Following these educational efforts evidence accumulated that changes in sexual behaviour, a reduction in the incidence of new HIV infections, and a reduction in the incidence of gonorrhoea had occurred in homosexual men. Unfortunately, some of these changes do not seem to have been sustained, particularly amongst young gay men.

After the government's health information campaigns in Britain in the 1980s, most people became aware of HIV/AIDS. But many seek more detailed information, particularly from health care staff. Some will be inappropriately anxious; others who are genuinely at high risk will need to obtain accurate information and personal advice. This presents an ideal opportunity for the clinician to practise preventive medicine and respond both sympathetically and with sound practical information.

Preventing sexual transmission

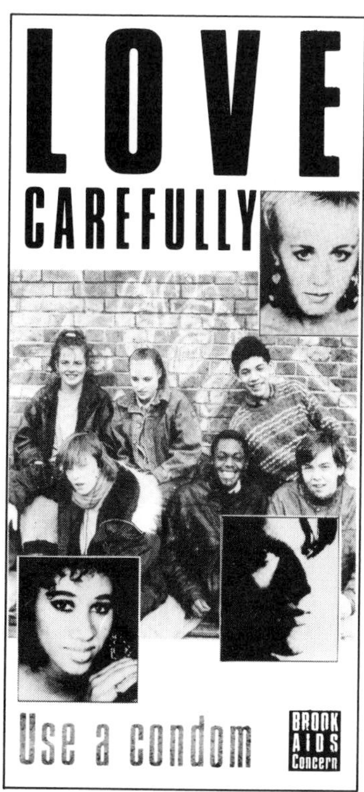

Advertisement for "safe sex".

As outlined in previous chapters, the epidemiology of HIV infection in the UK indicates that people who take part or have taken part in particular activities are currently at much higher risk than others. These people include homosexual and bisexual men, injecting drug users, haemophiliacs, the sexual partners of these individuals, and those who have had sexual contacts in parts of Africa and other parts of the world, such as south and south-east Asia, where heterosexual transmission predominates. Nevertheless, everyone is potentially at risk of infection. Even though the prevalence among those without a recognised risk factor is currently low, it requires sexual contact with only one infected person for transmission to occur. Those who are HIV seronegative and in a mutually monogamous relationship, have nothing to fear. The sensible message to everyone else must be: "To reduce your risk reduce your number of sexual partners, know about your partner's previous sexual and drug use history, and use a condom." Condoms may not provide total protection, but will substantially reduce risk if used properly and always. They therefore need to be available when needed, and it is worthwhile encouraging local chemists, pubs and clubs, and the local health authority to improve availability, as well as aiming to improve image and acceptability. Men and women can obtain condoms free of charge from family planning clinics and STD or departments of genitourinary medicine. Condoms should be used only with *water-based* lubricants (such as KY jelly). Oil-based lubricants can damage the rubber. Virucidal spermicides may offer additional protection but have not been fully evaluated *in vivo*. More recently, the female condom has become available providing further choice of methods for risk reduction.

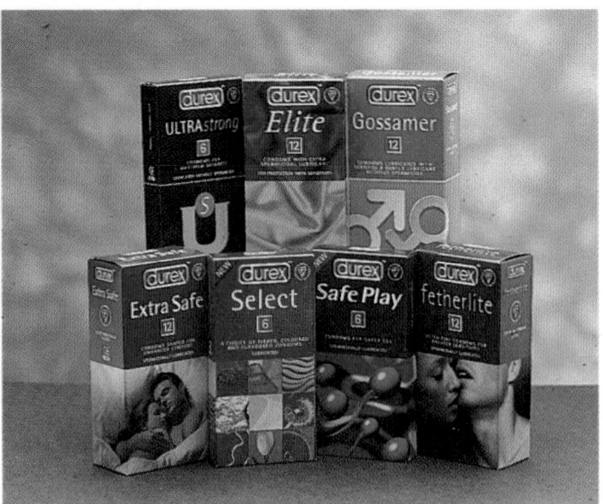

Reproduced with permission of Health Network.

When advice is being given to individuals, it is important to assess their risk factors for infection. If they are engaged in high risk activities safer sex needs to be emphasised strongly whether they are infected or not. Safer sex was discussed in the chapter on counselling. If uninfected, and still participating in high risk activities, the individual runs the risk of infection and, if infected, runs the risk of infecting others.

It is now felt that there are medical advantages (prophylaxis against *P. carinii* pneumonia, use of zidovudine, combination therapy and new protease inhibitor drugs, and monitoring of the immune system) to an individual knowing if they are positive. Disadvantages to being identified as positive have been covered earlier. STD clinics or departments of genitourinary medicine offer the opportunity to all patients to be tested. Testing can also be carried out by general practitioners and in antenatal clinics, with appropriate counselling to patients. Clinicians should be aware of the importance of assuring and maintaining confidentiality in testing patients for HIV. Whether the individual opts to take the test or not, advice should be given on risk reduction.

The HIV seropositive individual may consider bringing his or her sexual partner for counselling and the offer of testing. This and partner notification are best carried out by specially trained staff in STD clinics. Both men and women may want to know their status if for no other reason than to stop infecting others if antibody positive. Women may also be concerned to know their serological state because of the implications of a positive result for future pregnancies.

Advice to at-risk individuals

- Safer sexual practices
- Fewer partners, less risk
- Use condoms

Preventing transmission in those who inject drugs

Advice to injecting drug users

- If possible, stop injecting drugs
- If you must inject drugs, get your own works and don't share them
- Practise safer sex

Free booklets for at-risk individuals.

Preventing transmission of HIV among injecting drug users must rely on stopping the sharing both of needles and of other paraphernalia of drug use (syringes, mixing bowls, spoons, etc) used in injecting—"works"—as well as advising on safer sexual practices.

Users need to be advised of the risks of sharing works and that this applies to any injecting, whether intravenous, intramuscular, or subcutaneous ("skin popping"). Equally important is advice on the risks of transmitting or acquiring the virus sexually, as well as of the potential risks of both male and female prostitution, as this may be used to finance a drug habit. Evidence to date shows that drug users are beginning to accept safer injecting practices but have not changed their sexual behaviour to the same degree.

Ideally, the best primary prevention for drug users is to stop using drugs. Help can be sought from the local drug dependence services (if such exist) as well as from voluntary agencies—for example, Narcotics Anonymous—or from dialling the operator and asking for Freephone Drug Problems for a recorded message of how to locate local services.

If stopping is at present unrealistic the next option is to stop injecting and switch to sniffing, smoking, or swallowing drugs. Again drug advice agencies may be able to provide support. The role of oral methadone maintenance programmes in reducing HIV transmission risk is currently being evaluated.

If stopping injecting is not possible then stopping sharing must be the message for everyone. If this is the only realistic solution it is important that every injecting user has his or her own set of clean works. It is worth knowing which chemists in the area will sell needles and syringes. Needle exchange programmes have been set up throughout the UK and available evidence suggests these have had a useful role in reducing HIV transmission. Drug users must also have easy access to health information outside the formal health service structure.

As with those at risk from sexual transmission, anyone who is a drug user can be offered HIV antibody testing with appropriate counselling. It is essential that adequate support is available over the test period, as a positive result may precipitate a bout of chaotic drug using, putting both the client and others at risk. Whether testing takes place or not, advice on safer sex and condom use needs to be given as well as additional advice on contraception for women.

Preventing vertical transmission

> **Preventing vertical transmission**
>
> - Contraception advice for seropositive women
> - Offer counselling and ? HIV testing to pregnant women at high risk of infection
> - Offer ? termination of pregnancy to seropositive women
> - Seropositive mothers should avoid breastfeeding if possible

The risk of an HIV positive pregnant woman transmitting HIV to her unborn child is thought to be about 15% in developed countries, but is higher in developing countries (approximately 30%). Seropositive women or women who are considering parenthood with a seropositive man need to be counselled about the risks of infection in her unborn child. Primary prevention of pregancy entails providing adequate contraception *as well as* the use of a condom to prevent sexual transmission of HIV between partners. Unwanted pregnancy has resulted from couples switching from more reliable methods of contraception to condoms alone.

Women at high risk of infection should be offered counselling and HIV antibody testing if they want it in the early stages of pregnancy. If they take the test women should understand that if they are seropositive, therapeutic termination can be offered on grounds of risk to the fetus. Of course, the final informed decision must be taken by the mother whether to continue the pregnancy. A recent study has shown a marked reduction in vertical transmission if the mother is given zidovudine during pregnancy. This strategy is only affordable in the developed world. Seropositive women should also be advised against breastfeeding their infants, since the risk of transmission due to breastfeeding is estimated to be 14%. This advice may not be feasible in a developing country, however, where alternative forms of feeding may not be a practical option or medically advisable.

Preventing transmission by blood, blood products, and organ donation

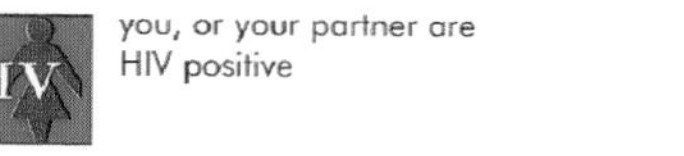

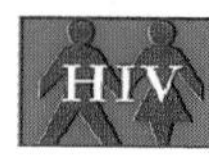

you, or your partner are HIV positive

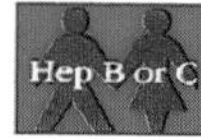

you carry the hepatitis B or C virus

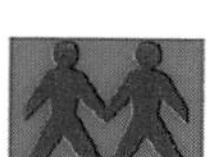
you are a man who has had sex with another man, even 'safe sex' using a condom

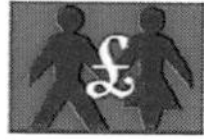
you have ever worked as a prostitute

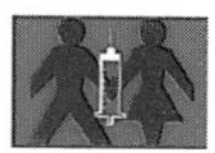
you have ever injected yourself with drugs, even once

You should not give blood FOR A YEAR after sex with:

a man who has had sex with another man (if you are female)

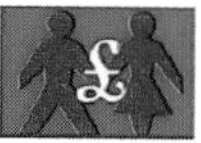
a prostitute

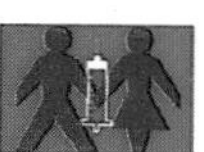
anyone who has injected themselves with drugs

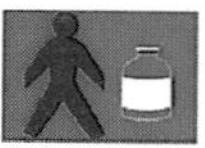
anyone with haemophilia or a related blood clotting disorder who has received clotting factor concentrates

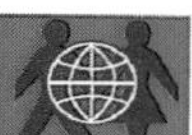
anyone, of any race, who has been sexually active in Africa* in the past year. This is because the main route of HIV infection there is heterosexual sex.

* apart from Morocco, Algeria, Tunisia, Libya or Egypt

Please do not give blood if you think you need a test for HIV or hepatitis, or if you have had sex in the past year with someone you think may be HIV or hepatitis positive.
If you have any doubts or questions, talk to the nurse or doctor.

Government advice to those who should not give blood. *Reproduced with permission from the Department of Health Publications.*

All blood transfusion centres give written instructions to potential donors not to give blood if they have a risk factor for infection with HIV. Those asked not to donate are shown in the table. They should also be advised not to donate semen and not to carry a donor card.

All blood donations in Britain have been screened for HIV antibody since the end of 1985. All suspected or confirmed positive blood is discarded. At present about 0·001% of donations are confirmed positive. There remains an extremely small risk of an infected but false negative sample being transfused. This risk is thought to be less than one per million donations.

All factor VIII for haemophiliacs is now heat treated to destroy any active virus.

Donors of all organs and semen must be screened for HIV antibody before organs are used.

Control of infection in the home and workplace has been discussed in an earlier chapter.

Foreign travel

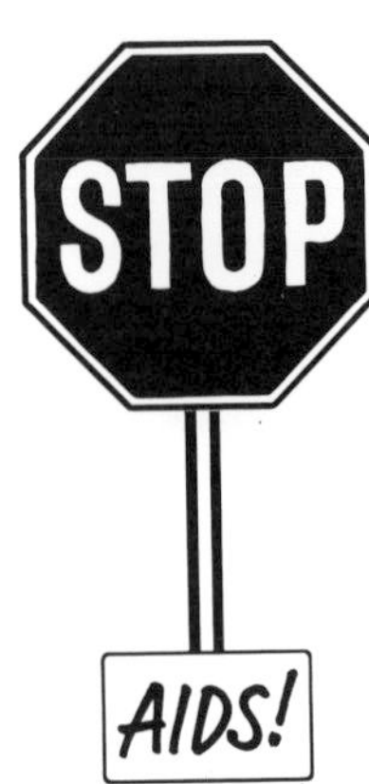

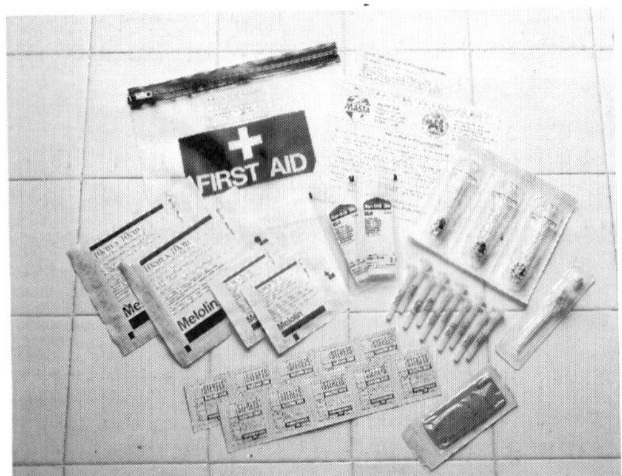

This sterile equipment pack is available from MASTA, London School of Hygiene and Tropical Medicine, Keppel St, London WC1E 7HT (tel. 0171 631 4408). It costs £13.50 incl. p&p.

When travelling abroad, as at home, everyone should be reminded of the risks of casual sexual encounters, particularly in areas where HIV is highly prevalent. In parts of the world, particularly in central Africa, south and south-east Asia, transmission of HIV is primarily by heterosexual activity. High rates of infection have been shown among the sexually active population of both sexes in some major cities, and infection rates are high in prostitutes. Causual heterosexual encounters are therefore very risky and are best avoided. The use of condoms may provide some protection from infection. In the United States, the highest rates of infection, as in the UK, are in homosexual men and drug users.

Travellers should be reminded that in many parts of the world screening of blood for HIV before blood transfusion is not carried out, and there is frequent reuse of needles and syringes for medical purposes.

The Medical Advisory Service for Travellers Abroad (MASTA) provides information for travellers and sells a sterile medical equipment pack containing disposable needles, intravenous cannulae, etc. They also supply emergency dental packs. Difficulties may arise if emergency blood transfusion is required. The local British embassy may be able to advise on availability of plasma expanders or on local donor panels.

Health professionals as health educators; surveillance and monitoring

Some sources of health education material and AIDS information

- Local health promotion department
- Local sexually transmitted diseases clinic
- National AIDS Helpline 0800 567123
- Health Education Authority, Hamilton House, Mabledon Place, London WC1H 9TX 0171 383 3833
- National AIDS Trust, New City Cloisters, 188/196 Old St, London EC1V 9FR 0171 814 6767
- The Terrence Higgins Trust, 52/54 Grays Inn Road, London WC1X 8JU Helpling 0171 242 1010 (noon to 10 pm every day)
- The Haemophilia Society, 123 Westminster Bridge Road, London SE1 7HR 0171 928 2020
- SCODA (Standing Conference on Drug Abuse), Water Bridge House, 32–36 Loman St, London SE1 0EE 0171 928 9500
- Cardiff AIDS Helpline (10 am to 10 pm Mon–Fri) 01222 223443
- Northern Ireland AIDS Line, Belfast (7.00 pm to 10 pm) Mon–Fri 01232 326117

Many health professionals may be asked to speak to other health and social services workers, to local schools or colleges, and may need appropriate information. The box gives a short list of useful contacts from which personal advice, and health education materials, including leaflets, videos, and teaching packs, can be obtained. Voluntary and pressure groups often offer a fund of information on local resources, as well as providing support for individuals. Health education messages need to be imaginative, comprehensive, and relevant to the group addressed. Advice from local health promotion officers and local groups is often essential in helping to get the appropriate message across. Prevention cannot be limited to health service settings and needs to include community work in pubs, clubs, and schools. Other strategies include the employment of "outreach workers", working outside the health care setting in close collaboration with voluntary groups, to contact, for example young people, drug users and women working as prostitutes.

The effectiveness of preventive strategies and estimates of the magnitude of the epidemic can be assessed only by continued monitoring of HIV infection rates and the occurrence of AIDS cases

All doctors are invited to participate in confidential reporting of cases of AIDS to the Communicable Disease Surveillance Centre (61 Colindale Avenue, London NW9 5EQ; tel 0181 200 6868). Public health service and other laboratories also report numbers and risk group of seropositive patients to Colindale.

Evaluation of health education strategies are being carried out through population studies of knowledge about AIDS, social studies of sexual and drug using behaviour, and seroprevalence studies in populations of both high and low risk.

A continued and coordinated national and international effort through education, surveillance, and research is required if we are to meet the public health challenge of AIDS.

17 BEING HIV ANTIBODY POSITIVE

Jonathan Grimshaw

I learned that I was HIV antibody positive late in 1984. There was, at that time, no formal counselling or organised psychological and social support for those discovering that they had been exposed to this newly identified virus.

The doctor who gave me the test result told me that I seemed the sort of person who would be able to cope and asked if I would be "all right". I, aware that he would be unable to help and therefore embarrassed if I said I couldn't cope, and not wanting to lose his good opinion of me, said "Yes, I'll be all right".

Initial reactions

Of course I couldn't cope. I was very frightened. I was convinced I was going to die and was afraid—not so much of death itself, but of the emotional and physical suffering that would precede it. I was 30 years old at the time; I had not experienced the death of anyone close to me and I was angry and utterly bewildered at having to confront it myself so soon.

I was also very alone. I knew no one in the same situation. Public fear of AIDS, and those perceived to be "AIDS carriers" was at its height and I was afraid that confiding in people, even those close to me, to ask for support or understanding, would invite rejection and hostility. On the other hand, knowing I had HIV changed me and my life fundamentally. Trying to conceal this from people, especially those close to me, meant I had to be dishonest and put up barriers which undermined the trust and openness on which my closest relationships were founded.

I also felt an overwhelming sense of loss. I felt that I no longer had any control over my own life. From now on, every aspect of existence would be determined by a virus. At that time safer sex, even in the gay community to which I belonged, was not the norm: to ask for safer sex was to risk advertising, or creating a suspicion, that one was infected. No one, I thought, would want to have a relationship with a person who had HIV. I thought I would never know sexual intimacy, or be loved, again. When I became ill I would lose not just my health but my income, my security, my independence, and my self-esteem. I realised how much of the "meaning" of one's own life—goals, aspirations, dreams, motivation, endurance, hope, fulfilment—depends on the unconscious assumption of a future. I had lost that too.

Because all this was too much to cope with, I was drunk or tranquillised for much of the time during the two months after diagnosis.

Self-help and professional help

At the end of 1984, the Terrence Higgins Trust set up the first support group for people who were HIV antibody positive. It gave me, and the others there, a safe environment in which to talk, openly and honestly, about what had happened to us and how we felt about it, to cry for what we had lost and to talk about our anger. Most importantly perhaps, it made us realise that we were not on our own and that the feelings we had been experiencing individually were not only felt by the others but were a natural reaction to the situation we were in.

The sense of anger that some of us had felt became, as we developed a shared understanding of it, translated into a determination to try to ensure that no one else should have to endure the sense of social and emotional isolation that we had experienced. That determination led to the establishment of Body Positive—the first self-help group in the UK, and perhaps in the world, for people with HIV.

The potential psychological and social impact of a positive HIV antibody test result are now well recognised and documented, as is the importance of referring those whose result is positive to counsellors and agencies equipped to provide the various forms of support and help that may be needed. Although individual circumstances will differ, many of the psychological and emotional needs are common to everyone faced with a life-threatening illness and forced to confront their own mortality.

There are, however, three particular aspects of HIV that make it, and the experience of living with it, different from other conditions: the fact that it is sexually transmissible, the stigma associated with it and the uncertainty of prognosis.

Sexual relationships

Not long after receiving my test result, I met someone who was himself untested and who became my partner for several years. My fears about never being loved again were unjustified. Since the relationship ended, however, the prospect of establishing another has become increasingly daunting. I am afraid to reveal that I am HIV antibody positive to a potential partner in case I'm rejected. If I don't reveal my HIV status at first, and a relationship develops, I risk rejection when eventually it becomes impossible to conceal.

Even casual sexual relationships are fraught with anxiety. Insisting on safer sex does not necessarily invite the suspicion it used to and health education campaigns on AIDS have emphasised that people have a responsibility to protect themselves. But I know from experience that it is impossible to be totally in control of an activity in which someone else is taking part. If unsafe sex does occur, I can say to myself intellectually that it was not totally my responsibility and that the other person would not have wanted it to happen unless he too was HIV antibody positive. Emotionally, however, I feel that knowing I have HIV gives me an extra responsibility and I could never forgive myself if someone became infected as a result of having sex with me. It seems easier to avoid the possibility altogether, although the cost, in terms of feelings of isolation and loss of self-worth, is sometimes almost unbearable.

Stigma and discrimination

Although public education has removed much of the fear and prejudice surrounding HIV and AIDS, it seems that the disease is irrevocably stigmatised. Even though surveys have shown a majority of people to have sympathetic and liberal attitudes towards people with HIV or AIDS, the same people believe that others are not sympathetic. The belief that the public is not sympathetic is most widely held amongst people with HIV or AIDS themselves. As a result, while perhaps relatively few people with HIV or AIDS have experienced discrimination or stigma, many fear it.

The fear of discrimination has, perhaps, a far greater impact on people with HIV than discrimination itself. It affects relationships, the choices one is able to make in life and one's self-esteem. I have experienced, and been hurt by, ignorance but don't think I have ever experienced what I would call discrimination. I will never know whether that is because of the restrictions I've placed on my life in order to avoid it.

Uncertainty

A few years ago my T4 helper cell count began a slow but continuous decline and I developed "shingles" which, at that time was thought to be indicative of HIV disease progression. Thinking that progression was now inevitable, although my doctor was reassuring me that the T4 helper cell count was still within "normal" range, I retired from work. Since then, my T4 helper cell count has improved and, well over a decade since my test result, I am still healthy.

No one can tell me now whether I am a "non-progressor" or a "slow-progressor" or whether I will develop AIDS within six months and be dead within a year. Having overcome the initial certainty of dying, I now face complete uncertainty. In some ways this is more difficult. I cannot "assume" a future for myself but somehow have to continue with my life. It is an exhausting paradox.

Most of my friends now are people who do not have HIV or are untested. The great majority of my friends with HIV have died. To many people I probably seem, and should consider myself to be, extremely fortunate. In some ways I am. Being forced to confront my own mortality made me think about the purpose of my life. If I was going to die, I needed to die knowing that I had, in my own terms, used my life well. Because of the way I have used my time since 1984, I can now do that. I have learned how to make myself happy, from day to day, by balancing hope and pessimism. There is an old Japanese saying that "to endure the unendurable is true endurance". It is an apt aphorism for living, continually, with HIV.

18 HAVING AIDS

Caroline Guinness

I was diagnosed in 1986 when there was very little knowledge of HIV. I had just been diagnosed as having precancer of the cervix, but I felt there was something else wrong—just an instinctive feeling—there was nothing in particular. So I went to my GP, and in fact saw a locum who was very young and enthusiastic. He felt my neck and said my glands were up, which I suppose alerted him to HIV, although he didn't say anything, suggesting it might be glandular fever. He took some blood, and said I should return three days later.

When I went back for the results he said they were negative for glandular fever, but that he had also requested an "AIDS test". I remember feeling really cold when he said that. I knew that maybe that was what it was, because two years beforehand, shortly after my husband left me and I was very vulnerable, I had slept with a bisexual man. I told the doctor that I thought he should have talked to me about it first, and that I wanted the test stopped. He said it was too late as it had already gone to the laboratories. I said in that case I didn't want to know what the result was.

About two weeks later, my own doctor who was back, just turned up at my house. He knew that I didn't want to know the result of the test, but he thought that, as an intelligent woman, I should know that it was positive. Even though I had some suspicions, I found that being told for definite was a different thing altogether. I went into shock. My first reaction was to ask how long I had to live, and he said probably about five years. My next thought was for my daughter, who was 3 years old at the time, and whether she would be infected too. The doctor didn't think there would be any risk to her as I had obviously contracted it after she was born, but I knew nothing about transmission or anything like that. He suggested another doctor at the practice who had more experience than him, and had been treating a couple of gay men, and that I should go and see her, which I did. She was really sweet, but she didn't know anything about other Genitourinary Medicine (GUM) clinics, voluntary agencies etc. On the other hand, she was good because she was a very firm believer in complementary therapies, so recommended vitamins and minerals and things which, looking back on it, was actually the best thing she could have done. But not having any counselling and not being in a specialist situation were not good. For the next six months or so I was just in denial—it hadn't sunk in at all. I didn't want to tell anybody because the atmosphere was really bad in those days, lots of scaremongering in the Press, calling it the "gay plague" etc.

I did tell a couple of close friends whom I lived with at the time. One, as a gay man, found it very ironical as he thought that if anyone should have tested positive it should have been him, and the other was a girlfriend of mine who sort of panicked. She was OK, but having lost her partner a couple of years before, she couldn't bear the thought of losing somebody else, which of course didn't help me. I didn't want anyone like Social Services to know, as Lee had just started nursery school, and I didn't want it getting out. So I just kept quiet and continued in my state of denial.

I couldn't cope with work at all—it seemed irrelevant. I told my colleagues that I needed treatment for my cervix which I thought might help explain my lack of concentration. Their reaction was that it wasn't such a big deal, and as I felt I couldn't tell them what was really happening, I resigned. That left me with financial problems, but I didn't want to go to Social Services because of Lee.

I had a partner at the time whom I had been with for six months before being diagnosed, and having to tell him, and him having to get tested was the other thing that was really frightening. Because I didn't know how to tell him, I asked my best friend, whom he got on very well with, if he would tell him. My partner thought that he was going to be told I wanted to split up, so when he realised what it actually was, his initial reaction was one of relief, but the following two weeks, while he got tested and waited for the results, were pretty fraught. We had no information about transmission, but luckily the test came back negative, which was a relief.

My fears about Lee being infected went on for quite some time because I felt I was not getting any real reassurance. I worried about things like her using my toothbrush, and I remembered I had cut my finger and she had helped me put the plaster on, and stuff like that. All those things kept going through my mind. The doctor I was seeing didn't recommend that I had her tested, as she firmly believed Lee would be alright. Looking back on it, I think that if I had just had her tested then I would have felt a lot more reassured, because the whole issue bugged me subconsciously for a long time.

Another very stressful event which happened that year was that a close friend of mine told me he had AIDS. He didn't want anybody to know, and he asked if myself and a couple of other friends could look after him. His health went downhill so quickly and he started getting dementia and incontinence etc, and for me it was like looking in a mirror—very frightening. He did actually go public in the end, but he died shortly before Christmas, so all in all it was quite a bad year.

In 1987, about a year after my diagnosis, through the Terrence Higgins Trust (THT) I finally found out about GUM clinics and I attended James Pringle House, Middlesex Hospital, which made a huge difference to me. I really wanted to meet other HIV positive women—I'd never met any, and still felt as if I was the only woman who had the virus. Someone at THT told me about a support group called Positively Women, who met once a week, so I went along to the group and met a couple of other positive women which helped a lot. I eventually became the Director of Positively Women, and the next three years were really hard work. There was nothing for women at all, so we tried to produce leaflets and information. Despite doing interviews and media work, I never went public about my HIV status. Although our slogan said "For positive women, run by positive women", people never seemed to twig with me; I think they had some vision of what someone with HIV should look like, which I didn't really fit into. Positive women were very much seen as drug users or prostitutes, and most of the women were keeping quiet, usually to protect their families. Through Positively Women, I did many hospital visits to AIDS wards and I used to find that stressful, worrying that I might catch something if I was going to see someone with meningitis or TB.

However, after three years my energy was beginning to dwindle, and I also felt I wasn't spending enough time with Lee, so in 1991, I resigned as the Director, and went part-time. It gave me a bit more time to myself, and because I felt so run down I started using complementary therapies such as acupuncture reflexology, which I'm still having, and which made a difference.

I continued to attend the clinic every three months for a regular follow-up, and the relationship I had with my doctor was very good. She trusted my own judgement on my health, and I found we could work together. She also understood my need for complementary therapies. Seeing the same people on each visit helped maintain continuity and build up a relationship, which was important.

I decided to tell my daughter when she was about 10 years old. She's very bright and reads the newspapers, and it seemed the right time for her. Although I had never gone public about it, I knew it was going to get out at some point, and I didn't want Lee to find out from anyone else. I thought Lee might suspect, but in fact she hadn't. Her first reaction when I told her was to burst into tears, and then she felt embarrassed about crying which made me feel awful as it was quite a natural reaction. For a week or so she kept asking me how I was, and if there was anything in particular that she could do to help. I said she could give me a hand with the housework, but that didn't last very long—I don't think that was what she was expecting! It became immediately apparent that there were no services for children, and she was desperate to meet other kids in the same situation. I suggested to Lee that she didn't tell any friends for a while until she got used to the fact. Anyway she did actually tell a schoolfriend who immediately told everyone else which was exactly what I didn't want to happen.

Her school had been helpful—I had spoken to the Head, her teacher, and the school counsellor before telling her, but she still needed to talk to a trained counsellor, and again she needed to meet other kids in the same situation. None of the organisations offered services for children, but I got a letter from a woman in a similar situation and we met up so that Lee could meet her daughter, which was good for both of them, and at least she knew she wasn't on her own. Lee also started seeing a child psychologist which she really benefited from and she still goes along there when she wants to, but nothing regular.

I think that over the last year or so my energy really hasn't been so good, and as Lee has now reached 13 and is going through everything that 13-year-olds do, I could really do with some help now. Her father was in Australia when I was diagnosed, and I didn't want to tell him by 'phone or letter, so I was hoping that he would be coming over to the UK at some point. Because I'd been told that I had about five years to live, I wanted to sort things out as quickly as possible. Anyway, he did come over and I told him, and he had a really odd reaction: he seemed to think I was trying to emotionally blackmail him, which really upset me. It was only later that I found out through a mutual friend that he felt that if he hadn't left me for someone else, I would never have slept with this bisexual man, and so he felt responsible, a thought which had never entered my head. His whole reaction was one of pure guilt, but then over the years that all changed, and for the last few years he's been really supportive.

At the beginning of 1992 I found I was pregnant, and I decided I wanted a termination, and that at the same time I wanted to be sterilised as I didn't want to go through this worry again. I knew enough about transmission at that point to know there was a 10–15% chance that I could pass the virus on, and although that's quite a low risk, I had seen enough other women take the chance and go through the whole nine months and following 18 months not knowing whether the child was infected or not, and I felt I didn't have that in me. I was referred to a hospital and I went there and saw a doctor in outpatients. She knew nothing about HIV—absolutely nothing. She automatically assumed I would want a termination, and before she examined me she removed all the blankets and coverings from the table, so again obviously had no idea about transmission or anything. She also asked the nurse what precautions she should be taking in front of me. It made me feel awful at what was a traumatic time anyway.

About a month ago I was involved in a conference called Living Proof, the first conference for long-term survivors ever, which was really illuminating and quite empowering. There were a lot of other women there which was great to see. I went to three workshops during the two-day event and it was amazing how the experiences of both women and men were so similar. We had all been told first that we probably had five years, then seven years, then 10 years etc. Although my Consultant never said this, it had been the general consensus, and the type of the thing you read in the press, so that when you go past those dates you feel more and more isolated. When you have also suffered so much loss and lost so many people on the way, there is a tinge of guilt that you are still here. Friends whom I told originally have sort of forgotten about it now because it's been going on for so long and they don't seem to realise that I'm still going through it all, and that it takes a large chunk out of my life, that I had to resign my job and go onto benefits.

You feel that people are waiting for you to die. It's still the uncertainty of just not knowing, constantly trying not to be in denial, because there've been enough people I know who have had the virus longer than I have and have died, and I do have definite symptoms. If I was in America I would have been diagnosed as having AIDS a while ago because my CD4 count has been hopping between 150–200 over the last two years. Luckily they don't do that here, because psychologically that's a hard one.

When I was admitted into hospital last year, the doctor was trying to be reassuring, saying that it wasn't necessarily HIV-related, but I didn't believe it. I found that most of the nurses had had no specialist training which made me feel a bit vulnerable. One morning I woke to find a young agency training nurse looking at my file; she said, "Oh, you were diagnosed in 1986 and you're still alive—that's amazing", and I thought "I just don't need this, I really don't." I was feeling so ill and didn't really have the strength to deal with it.

When you live in a little closed society like I do medically, where you go into a clinic, where everybody is wonderful and the service is fantastic, you forget about the lack of knowledge and the attitudes outside that world.

INDEX